PARENTING

ADHD

A New Approach to Understanding and Parenting Your ADHD Child

Rebecca Miller

© Copyright 2020 by Rebecca Miller - All rights reserved.

The content contained within this book may not be reproduced, duplicated or transmitted without direct written permission from the author or the publisher.

Under no circumstances will any blame or legal responsibility be held against the publisher, or author, for any damages, reparation, or monetary loss due to the information contained within this book. Either directly or indirectly.

Legal Notice:

This book is copyright protected. This book is only for personal use. You cannot amend, distribute, sell, use, quote or paraphrase any part, or the content within this book, without the consent of the author or publisher.

Table of Contents

Introduction 6

Chapter 1 – Understanding ADHD 8

    What Causes ADHD? 8

    Symptoms of ADHD 11

    Is it Really ADHD? 19

    What to Expect if your Child has ADHD? 21

    Complications 25

Chapter 2 – Diagnosing ADHD 31

    Sets up an initial meeting 33

    Preparing for the ADHD Screening 38

    What to Expect from the ADHD Assessment or Screening? 40

    Some Diagnosis Tips 48

    How Long Does it Take to Get the Results? 53

Chapter 3 – Managing Life with ADHD 63

    Build structure and set routines at home 71

    Other Do's and Don'ts when Parenting a Child with ADHD at Home 84

    Managing your Child's ADHD at School 92

Work together with your child's teacher 98

Create and implement a behavior plan 103

Chapter 4 – Medications for ADHD 136

Stimulant Medications 137

Non-stimulant Medications 139

Alternative Medicines and Treatments 144

Coping and Proper Support 146

Conclusion 147

Introduction

The life of a parent with a kid suffering from ADHD (attention deficit hyperactivity disorder) can be extremely challenging and frustrating. If you are a parent to an ADHD child then you may get overwhelmed with all the difficult challenges that you might be facing. However, note that you can make the whole process of caring for and parenting a child with such a condition easier and more manageable.

One thing that you can do is to be as educated about ADHD as possible. That way, you can be a big help to your child in overcoming his/her daily challenges. You will know exactly how you can channel your child's excess energy into positive areas while bringing calmness to the entire family. Your knowledge about ADHD will also help you address the problems exhibited by your child as early and consistently as possible. With that, you can play a major role in his success regardless of his condition.

To inform parents of kids suffering from ADHD is the ultimate goal of this book. This is why this book was created, to shed light on the condition and help parents deal with their children's condition every step of the way. Through this book, you will become more familiar with ADHD and the different ways you can help your child cope with it. In the end, you will become a more empowered and stronger parent, lending a hand to your child no matter how difficult his condition is.

Chapter 1 – Understanding ADHD

ADHD, which is the acronym for attention deficit hyperactivity disorder, is a medical condition characterized by a sufferer's difficulty when it comes to paying attention and controlling impulsive behaviors. A person who suffers from this condition may experience restlessness, causing him/her to be constantly active. ADHD is also characterized by certain differences in brain activities and development that might affect the sufferer's ability to focus, control himself, or sit still.

If you have a child with this condition then this might greatly affect him at home and school and when it comes to building relationships. ADHD is a very frustrating and challenging condition considering its major impact on a child's life, especially during his formative years.

What Causes ADHD?

As a neurological condition that has a major impact on the focus and attention of kids and adults suffering from it, ADHD's treatment requires a full understanding of what specifically causes it in the first place. As a parent, you surely want to know what triggers your child to experience the symptoms of ADHD. Knowing the cause of this condition can help you identify the most appropriate way to treat your child's case.

Here are just some of the most common ADHD causes and risk factors:

- **Some problems with pregnancy** – Kids born prematurely or those who have low birth weights are at risk of developing ADHD. The same risk is exhibited by children whose mothers experienced risky and difficult pregnancies.

  Women who did not stop drinking alcohol and smoking during the time they are pregnant are also prone to giving birth to a child suffering from ADHD. Furthermore, kids with injured frontal lobe found in the brain, which controls emotions and impulses, may also deal with the neurological condition.

- **Heredity and genes** – This condition also seems to run in the family. This means that a child is most likely to develop ADHD if his parents or any of his close family also suffer from it. In some cases, both the child and his parent are even diagnosed with the condition at the same time.

- **Brain structure and function** – Another thing to take note of regarding the causes of ADHD is that those suffering from it have some notable differences in their brain structures and functions from those who do not have the condition.

  Studies that involve brain scans even showed that certain brain areas are either smaller or larger in ADHD sufferers than those without it. It was also identified that ADHD sufferers have an imbalance in their brain's neurotransmitter levels. There is also a high chance that such chemicals do not function properly.

While no one can pinpoint what is the exact cause of ADHD, the ones mentioned are known to be among the most common triggers. There is also a high likelihood of a child developing ADHD with constant exposure to environmental toxins, like lead. Specific groups of people also display a high risk of suffering from the condition, including those who have epilepsy and brain damage that happened while in the womb or because of a severe head injury during his childhood or adulthood.

Also, contrary to what other parents believe, ADHD has no connection whatsoever to consuming excessive amounts of sugar or too much exposure to television.

Symptoms of ADHD

How do you know if your child is suffering from ADHD and not just a normal bout of hyperactivity? Note that children are naturally hyperactive, so parents might get confused if their child's hyperactivity is normal or already a symptom of the neurological condition.

With that in mind, it helps to gather as much information as you can about the usual signs and symptoms of ADHD to avoid getting misled. Through this, you can act on the problem if it is indeed serious. Another thing to take note of is that those who suffer from ADHD have neurotransmitters (brain chemicals) that seem to function differently.

Sufferers also exhibit major differences in the manner through which their nerve pathways function. Now on to the symptoms - here are just a few of those that you have to watch out for. If your child exhibits most of them then maybe it is time to seek a pediatrician's help to have a correct diagnosis.

Hyperactivity

Hyperactivity is an obvious symptom of ADHD. The problem with this is that you might have a hard time distinguishing whether your child is just naturally active or if his hyperactivity is already a sign of the condition. This is the main reason why you should watch your child closely. In most cases, children who display the hyperactive symptoms of ADHD are always on the move.

For instance, your child may do a lot of things all at once, causing him to bounce from one activity to another. You may notice him having difficulty sitting still even if you force him to do so. If you were able to force him to sit, expect him to do so while still displaying other movements, like drumming his fingers, tapping his foot, or shaking his legs.

Also, observe whether your child's hyperactivity is accompanied by:

- Squirming and fidgeting even when sitting
- Frequently getting up to walk or run around

- Climbing or running excessively even in inappropriate times – This symptom is characterized in teens as restlessness.
- Excessive talking
- Difficulties doing his hobby or playing quietly
- Problems calming down or relaxing
- Exhibits a short fuse or quick temper
- Tends to get bored easily
- Commits careless mistakes
- Rushes through things
- Acts in a way that seems to disrupt others

It is important to note that hyperactivity in ADHD sufferers tends to vary based on age. For instance, toddlers and those who are in preschool-age seem to be always in motion. They even tend to jump on furniture. In most cases, preschoolers experience problems taking part in activities that require them to be in a group and sit still. It may even be difficult for them to listen to stories.

The same habits are also often displayed by school-age kids, although they display those less frequently. You may see them experiencing difficulties remaining seated. They may also fidget, talk excessively, and squirm. In both teens and adults, hyperactivity may be exhibited as restlessness. It might also be difficult for them to do activities quietly and calmly that involve sitting.

Inattention

This is another group or category of symptoms exhibited by ADHD sufferers. If your child has ADHD, then he may display inattention often characterized by his inability to focus. However, this does not necessarily mean that kids with ADHD can't focus or pay attention entirely. If you get them to do things or listen to topics they enjoy and are interested in, you can expect them to stay on the task and focus.

The problem is that when you give them tasks that they find boring or repetitive, they tend to tune those out immediately. The inattention symptom might also cause your child suffering from ADHD to experience difficulty staying on track. There is a great chance for him to bounce from one task to another without actually completing any. In some cases, he may also skip vital steps and procedures when performing a task.

The fact that your child is suffering from ADHD may also cause him to have a difficult time organizing his schoolwork and managing his time. He may have trouble focusing and concentrating especially if some things seem to go around him. For him to stay focused, you need to let him do certain activities in a quiet and calm environment.

To recap clearly, here are just some of the inattention symptoms that your child might display if he has ADHD:

- Trouble concentrating or remaining focused on a task – This means he easily gets bored or distracted even before he completes a task.

- Looks like he is not listening when you are talking to him

- Trouble following instructions and remembering things – It could be because he has a hard time paying attention to details.

- Often commits careless mistakes

- Often misplaces or loses certain items, like toys, books, and homework

- Problems remaining organized and finishing projects

- Can't plan ahead

- Inability to sustain attention when playing or doing certain activities and tasks
- Hesitates, dislikes, or prevents engaging in activities and tasks that need sustained mental effort, like homework and schoolwork

Impulsiveness

Your child may also be suffering from ADHD if you can no longer consider his impulsiveness as normal. The problem with this impulsiveness is that this might trigger issues with self-control. His impulsiveness might cause him to censor himself less compared to other kids. This results in him interrupting conversations, making tactless comments and observations, asking overly personal and irrelevant questions, and invading the space of others.

You may also have a difficult time instructing him to wait a bit or be patient. In most cases, your child may overreact to things emotionally. He may also be moodier compared to the others. This might result in others perceiving your child as not only weird but also needy and disrespectful. To ensure that you are helping in diagnosing your child's condition correctly, find out if his impulsiveness is characterized by the following:

- Acts or behaves without thinking
- Interferes with the games and conversations of others
- Makes predictions, instead of spending time-solving a problem
- Provides answers in class even when not called and without hearing the entire question
- Interrupts others
- Tends to say the wrong things at an inappropriate time
- Can't control powerful emotions, causing temper tantrums and angry outbursts
- Exhibits impatience most of the time
- Inability to wait for the right time to react or talk
- Has addictive tendencies
- Acts spontaneously or recklessly without considering consequences

- Has a hard time acting in a socially acceptable manner, like sitting still when attending a long meeting

Forgetfulness and Disorganization

ADHD might also make the life of your child become more chaotic and seem to be beyond his control, especially as he grows to adulthood. He may struggle with staying organized and keeping track of things. It might also be hard for him to sort out relevant information for a specific task, prioritize his to-do list, manage his time, and monitor his duties and responsibilities. It might be because he may also display the symptoms of forgetfulness and disorganization, leading to other issues, like:

- Poor organizational and time management skills, causing a cluttered and messy room, desk, or home
- Prone to procrastinating
- Chronic lateness
- Problems starting and completing tasks and projects
- A tendency to misplace or lose things, like phone, wallet, documents, and keys

- Inability to keep up with deadlines, commitments, and appointments due to forgetfulness

- A tendency to underestimate the required time to finish a particular task

Emotional Struggles

The problem with ADHD is that it can also result in serious emotional struggles. It is because its sufferers will struggle to manage and control their emotions and feelings, like frustration and anger. This is the main reason why your child might also show emotional symptoms of ADHD, including short and explosive temper, irritability, a high risk of getting stressed out or flustered easily, insecurity or low self-esteem, hypersensitivity to criticism, and issues with retaining motivation.

Is it Really ADHD?

However, take note that just because your child displays the symptoms mentioned above, especially the ones that fall under hyperactivity, impulsivity, and inattention, it does not necessarily point to ADHD right away. It is important to check whether the signs your child show still fall under what is normal. Also, find out if there are other stressful life events, psychological issues, and medical conditions with almost similar symptoms as ADHD that he is suffering from.

Furthermore, take note that before getting an accurate ADHD diagnosis, it is necessary to visit a mental health professional. The help of this professional is crucial in exploring and ruling out other possibilities that might be causing the symptoms, including learning disabilities (ex. issues with writing, language, reading, and motor skills), traumatic experiences or major life changes, and psychological conditions, like bipolar disorder, depression, and anxiety.

Your chosen mental health professional can also determine if the symptoms are caused by other behavioral disorders, like oppositional defiant, reactive attachment, and conduct disorders. You may also want to visit a doctor to find out if your child has other medical conditions, like epilepsy, sleep disorders, neurological disorders, and thyroid problems that also cause the symptoms.

If other mental and health issues were ruled out, though, and you were able to confirm that your child has ADHD, don't fret. While it is true that the symptoms mentioned earlier can disrupt your child's quality of life, there is still a way to manage them. Just talk to the right medical professional and have his entire condition assessed.

Also, take note that various health care and medical professionals may also have different diagnosis and means of supervising treatment for an ADHD patient. This is why you have to find out who among them truly suits what your child needs. Make sure that you look for a healthcare provider with enough experience and training when it comes to caring for kids with ADHD.

What to Expect if your Child has ADHD?

While ADHD has a lot of negative connotations, keep in mind that there are some good things that your child can get from having the condition. Yes, you need to act on it, so you and your kid will have a smooth-sailing life together but this does not necessarily mean that you have to stress yourself out or get overly depressed just because your child is diagnosed with ADHD.

It is also true that this condition can affect his ability to control his behavior, pay attention, and focus. However, take note that ADHD will also cause your child to show some positive qualities and strengths. Here are just some of the positive qualities and effects of this condition on your child as he grows up:

- **Energetic** – If properly managed, the almost unlimited amount of energy that your child has will allow him to be successful in various fields. He can always channel his energy towards activities that can make him successful in school, sports or playing field, and work.

- **Spontaneous** – Some ADHD sufferers were able to transform their impulsive behaviors into spontaneity. This is a good thing because this allows them to be more open and adventurous. Expect your child, therefore, to have the willingness to break free from what is deemed normal by trying new things. His spontaneity may also cause him to become the life and heart of a party.

- **Creative** – Being diagnosed with ADHD can also have a positive effect on your child, especially in terms of creativity. It is because his condition might cause him to have another perspective about life. With that, he will most likely approach certain situations and tasks with thoughtfulness and creativity. This quality is one of the main reasons why there are ADHD sufferers known for being inventive thinkers.

- **Compassionate** – The fact that they feel different makes some ADHD sufferers more compassionate than others who do not have the condition. In most cases, they seem to root for the underdogs. They are also willing to share their unconditional love to those who struggle.

- **Flexible** – If your child has ADHD, then expect him to be flexible. It is because he will most likely consider several options all at once. His condition does not cause him to just set himself on a single alternative. He will most likely open himself up to different ideas, which allows him to find the best solution to a particular problem.

- **Enthusiastic** – Your child's condition will hone his lively personality. Note that most ADHD patients are rarely boring. You can see them having an interest in several different things, leading to the development of their lively personalities. With that, expect your child to be fun and exciting to be with.

- **Strong drive and focus** – Channeled correctly, the strong drive and focus of your ADHD child can make him successful. Expect him to be more motivated than the others, whether it is at school, sports, or work. He will most likely strive to succeed.

  Furthermore, their strong drive and focus will prevent them from getting distracted when doing a task that they love. Once you give him an interesting task, he will be able to focus on it whether it is a hands-on or interactive activity.

See? Having ADHD is not a bad thing. However, despite the many positive qualities and effects of ADHD, it is still important to manage your expectations. Remember the complications and negative effects of ADHD on your child's life in their entirety so you can respond to them the right way.

Prepare for difficulties and challenges along the way, especially while you are still trying to figure out what will bring out the best in your child with ADHD. But just hang on tight there because eventually, you will learn how to be a good parent to your child, even with his condition. You will be able to find the most suitable coping method for him, too.

Complications

Even with the positive effects of ADHD, it is still advisable for parents to learn a thing or two about how to make their child cope with the disorder. It is because if left untreated or unmanaged, it can lead to a wide range of negative effects and complications. One of the negative effects of the condition is the higher risk of those suffering from it to experience academic failures and problems.

It is also normal for kids with the disorder to have low self-esteem and confidence, causing issues not only at school but also in building relationships. If you do not learn a few techniques in managing the symptoms of the disorder, then your child will also be more vulnerable to dealing with accidents because of his impulsiveness and somewhat incessant movements.

ADHD may also make it hard for children to interact in a social setting. Expect conversations to seem erratic for your child. Furthermore, he might battle following a storyline plus he tends to cut in the conversations or interrupt someone who is talking. The inability to control impulses might also make your child prone to drug and alcohol abuse as he is growing up.

Other complications that might come up because of ADHD, especially as your child grows into adulthood include:

- Poor performance not only in school but also in the workplace
- Financial troubles
- Unemployment
- Legal troubles/issues
- Frequent accidents
- Poor self-image
- Poor mental and physical health
- Unstable relationships
- Suicidal attempts

Aside from the mentioned complications, untreated ADHD may also put your child at risk of developing other psychological and development problems. If you do not try to do something to help your child with ADHD then he will also be prone to having any of these conditions:

Mental and physical health conditions

Some of the signs and symptoms of ADHD might cause the sufferer to develop various health conditions, like anxiety, compulsive eating, low self-esteem, chronic tension and stress, and substance abuse. He might also be at risk of neglecting vital checkups and medical instructions. Your child will be prone to forgetting the time he should take his medications and skipping his doctor's appointments.

Mood disorders

ADHD might also contribute to the development of various mood disorders, especially once your child reaches adulthood. Among the conditions affecting the mood that might be brought up by ADHD are bipolar disorder and depression. While you cannot point the exact cause to ADHD, note that repeated patterns of frustrations and failures caused by the disorder might worsen depression and mood disorders.

Severe anxiety

Anxiety disorders frequently happen to adults suffering from ADHD. The problem with this is that it can trigger extreme nervousness, worries, and other related symptoms that might overwhelm your child. The setbacks and challenges brought on by having ADHD might also worsen anxiety so make sure that you are with your child every step of the way while he is trying to recover from the disorder.

Learning disabilities

Your child might also have a lower score on academic tests than what is expected for his education, intelligence, and age. Because of your child's learning disabilities, he may also have problems communicating with and understanding others.

Financial and work difficulties

As your child grows into adulthood, he may suffer from career struggles and difficulties. He may also feel like he is an underachiever. These unwanted feelings and struggles might cause him to experience problems keeping a job, meeting deadlines, following the 9-to-5 routine, and adhering to corporate rules. He might also experience issues with financial management. You will see him struggling with late fees, excessive debt because of impulsive buying and spending, lost paperwork, and unpaid bills.

Relationship problems

Your child's relationships, whether it's for family, romance, or work, will also suffer if he does not know how to manage ADHD symptoms. The disorder might cause him to get easily fed up when a loved one constantly nags him to get organized, listen, or clean up. It might also strain his relationships with others, especially if those around him resent him for his insensitivity and irresponsibility.

Other psychiatric disorders

Apart from the ones mentioned, your child will also be prone to developing other psychiatric disorders. These include substance use disorders, personality disorders, and intermittent explosive disorders.

Dealing with the Complications

ADHD is indeed a condition with wide-reaching effects on various aspects of your child's life. It might lead to frustration, loss of confidence, embarrassment, disappointment, and hopelessness. The problem is your child is not the only one who will suffer. Seeing him that way, you may also feel hopeless. There is a tendency for you to feel hurt by the negative effects of ADHD on your child, especially if you see him having a difficult time controlling his life and fulfilling his potential.

This is the reason why you have to learn as much as you can about ADHD and how to cope with the complications. If your child displays most of the symptoms then the best way to deal with the complications is to visit a doctor right away. Your goal here is to get a correct and proper diagnosis. Do not be afraid if the diagnosis points out to ADHD.

Getting the diagnosis can even be a huge source of hope and relief for both you and your child. It is because this will let you understand the condition for the first time and how you can deal with it. Also, remember that whatever challenges your child experiences, it is not because he is flawed or weak. It is because he is a victim of attention deficit hyperactivity disorder. The good news is that there is hope since you and your child can work together to cope with or manage its negative effects.

Chapter 2 – Diagnosing ADHD

Now that you know the basics of ADHD, it is time to learn more about how to evaluate your child to determine if he indeed has the disorder. Remember that most of the symptoms of ADHD, like hyperactivity and problems with focus and concentration, are easy to confuse with other medical issues and disorders, like emotional problems and learning disabilities.

This means that just because of the symptoms that your child displays seem like he has ADHD, it does not instantly mean that he has the condition. To ensure that you evaluate him correctly, it would be best to get a thorough assessment and correct diagnosis. The whole ADHD evaluation process views several factors, including how much the symptoms displayed by your child affect his daily and school life.

Also, your child must meet a few criteria before getting diagnosed with ADHD. One more thing that you have to remember when evaluating your child is that several specialists and professionals are capable and qualified to perform the evaluation and diagnosis. Some of them are psychologists, psychiatrists, neurologists, psychotherapists, and pediatricians.

Before you book a meeting or appointment, ask whether your chosen healthcare provider is experienced when it comes to ADHD diagnosis. You can't expect your family doctor to be able to do a more detailed ADHD evaluation but you can ask for a referral whom you can contact to adequately examine and evaluate your child. Some general practitioners and pediatricians are also capable of diagnosing ADHD.

If your pediatrician suspects that your child is suffering from ADHD, then you can always request for a referral so you can work with a specialist who can perform further screening and evaluation. Another thing to remember is that it is not possible to diagnose the condition online, though you can find several online questionnaires and quizzes that are extremely useful if you want to screen your child yourself.

By taking the quizzes based on the condition of your child, you will have more confidence knowing that you can seek the help of the correct health professional who can give you a formal and correct diagnosis. Another thing to remember is that regardless of the kind of specialist who does the evaluation, the whole process still needs to include a few important things.

Here are just some of the things that your chosen specialist should do during a complete ADHD evaluation and assessment.

Sets up an initial meeting

The first thing that you can expect the specialist to do is to set up a meeting with both you and your child. This serves as a fact-finding meeting with the main goal of identifying the challenges, weaknesses, and strengths of your child. Expect the specialist to gather facts and information regarding certain life situations that have a huge impact on your child. These situations could be at school, home, or the community.

The specialist will also request more detailed information about your own and your child's health, whether it is in the past or present. Some of these include issues that you experienced during your pregnancy as well as when you gave birth. Your chosen specialist may also try to gather information about:

- Developmental milestones
- Early infancy
- Appetite

- Allergies
- Weight and height
- Sleep patterns
- Ongoing medical or development problems
- History of hospitalizations

Gathers information about the way your child functions

The specialist will also start looking into the challenges and struggles of your child, especially in three main or key areas – school, home, and social settings or relationships. During this stage, make sure to open up about the passions, interests, and strengths of your child, instead of just his weaknesses and struggles.

Makes use of normed ADHD rating scales

These rating scales refer to questionnaires you need to fill out. In most cases, the questionnaires will focus on gathering information about the difficulties your child experiences when doing his daily and school functions. After collecting the information, the specialist will then compare the results with the common behaviors displayed by other kids of the same age. Expect the specialist to do other behavioral assessments to evaluate ADHD, too.

Evaluates previous and current school performances

A good specialist will also evaluate the standardized tests and report cards of your child. He may also ask the present teacher of your child to fill out a rating scale. Furthermore, the specialist will ask about the additional help and support your child is receiving in terms of academics. Among these are class support and tutorials. All these details will be used in reviewing and evaluating the academic performance of your child.

Checks info based on the official criteria for ADHD diagnosis

Note that several factors and criteria should be present when diagnosing ADHD. The official criteria consist of nine kinds of attention problems and another nine impulsivity and hyperactivity symptoms. If your child is less than 16 years old and displays at least six of the problems on each list then he could be diagnosed with ADHD.

For children older than 16 years, checking at least five problems on each list will diagnose them with ADHD. The problems, however, should significantly affect the way your child functions. When checking the criteria, the evaluator should also consider other challenges apart from ADHD, including mental health issues, such as depression and anxiety, as well as learning differences.

It is because such challenges might co-occur with attention deficit hyperactive disorder or happen by themselves. If your chosen specialist is not qualified to examine such disorders or challenges for you then consider asking for a referral from him.

Sets up a follow-up meeting

A good specialist will also set up another meeting to check the results. If your child is positive for ADHD then expect this follow-up meeting to also discuss potential treatments, including ADHD medication and therapy (ex. cognitive behavioral therapy). You and the specialist will also discuss the support that your child needs at school as well as the changes in routines that you have to do at home together with the entire family.

Creates a plan to keep track of progress

You know that you are working with a reliable specialist for ADHD if he develops a good plan designed to monitor the treatment and find out if the changes in routines and the support received by your child are working. This is also the time to figure out whether it is necessary to make changes to the plan.

If your child is required to take ADHD medication then he needs to visit the clinic regularly. This is a huge help in allowing the prescriber to see whether the medication's dosage is safe and effective and if it has any side effects. Keeping track of progress is also essential in determining whether fine-tuning the treatments are necessary. To monitor everything, a medication log for ADHD is a must.

How to Diagnose ADHD?

With the help of your chosen specialist or doctor who has to do all the things mentioned above for him to evaluate your child's case correctly, ADHD diagnosis screening or tests will take place. In this case, your child will need to undergo a full physical exam. This includes hearing and vision screenings. To give a proper diagnosis, expect the doctor to begin asking questions regarding your child's health, activities, and behaviors.

After gathering all the required information, your doctor will confirm that your child indeed has ADHD if clear scenarios are showing his hyperactivity, impulsivity, and distractibility that go over what is normal for kids his age. Your doctor will also diagnose a child with ADHD if all these situations are present:

- The signs, symptoms, and ADHD behaviors started even when he was still young.

- His impulsive and hyperactive nature and distractibility greatly affect his life both at home and at school.

- A health examination confirms that no other learning or health issue causes the symptoms.

Preparing for the ADHD Screening

Before your first appointment with the doctor, expect to receive a few questionnaires and behavioral checklists that you need to answer. Make sure to complete these before going to your first meeting with your child's specialist. The forms that you have to answer will contain general information not only about your child but also the family. It will also contain information about the behavioral, medical, and developmental history of your child.

Make sure to prepare all these completed forms then bring these to your first appointment with the doctor. Apart from that, it is also advisable to collect and prepare these items and bring them during the evaluation. It is because most of these items are essential in ensuring that the doctor will make an accurate judgment.

- Medical records of your child
- Your contact details as well as the contact info of your child's pediatrician
- Contact details and names of teachers and other adults who play supervisory roles in your child's life, like those who are part of after-school programs.
- Prior test results, like personality assessments, achievement tests, and IQ tests – If he underwent ADHD evaluations in the past, make sure to bring the results, too. Include the names and contact details of the people who gave the tests and assessments.
- Your child's notes and report cards from school
- Insurance information

- Completed prep work for the parent interview
- Individualized education plans, if there are any

You may also need to make a written consent that you will give the doctor so he can contact the names you provided.

What to Expect from the ADHD Assessment or Screening?

The ADHD assessment or screening may take around 2-3 hours. This might go longer than that if the doctor feels the need to do psychological or educational tests. Though, the screening consists of the following vital components:

Parent Interview

This forms a vital part of the assessment. Here, the doctor will ask questions about the symptoms displayed by your child that somewhat point to ADHD. You will also be asked about its specific impact on the life of your child. There are also rating scales and checklists regarding the behavior of your child that you have to fill up. Both parents should get involved in filling up the forms and the actual interview.

To prepare for the parent interview, create a list of the specific concerns that you have about your child. Also, be prepared for all the possible questions that the medical specialist will throw at you. Among the most frequently asked questions during the parent interview are:

- When did the symptoms or issues start?

- Where and when do the symptoms and issues occur frequently? Is it at school, home, community, neighborhood, or during after-school activities? Does it usually happen when he is around his peers?

- How long is your child displaying the symptoms?

- Do the symptoms or problems take place more frequently? Do they occur to the point that is no longer normal in kids his age?

To be fully prepared for the interview, it is advisable to talk to his teachers and list down their related observations. Also, take note that while the doctor will evaluate and review your provided medical records, there is also a great chance that he will talk about the medical history of your child.

He may ask you several questions regarding your child's medical history, including:

- Do you have a family history of behavioral disorders and issues?

- Did your child suffer from a severe illness in the past? How did you manage it?

- Did you encounter problems or challenges during pregnancy?

- Did your child experience seizures, head injury, or headaches? If yes, then make sure to provide specific details regarding those cases.

- Has your child ever experienced stool soiling or bedwetting?

Apart from that, be prepared to share family issues that might have a major impact on your child. It is because your chosen medical professional might also ask you these questions during the interview:

- Are there any major changes in your family that happened recently? Some examples of these are having a newborn, moving into a new house, and transferring into a new school.

- Does anyone in your family suffer from a health issue?

- Did your family experience a loss recently, like the death of a loved one or pet?

- Is there chronic tension or discord within the family recently?

Even if you think that the whole ADHD assessment will focus on the frustrations and problems experienced by your child, it is still crucial to create a list of the strengths of your child. You should give this list to the doctor as this can provide him with a well-rounded perspective about what your child is experiencing.

Also, do not hesitate to share anything with the doctor. You may think that some issues are harder and more sensitive to tackle while others are not that relevant. Still, it is advisable to not leave anything out no matter how you think it is irrelevant. Note that the specialist will be the one to decide which one plays a major role in the behavior of your child, so make sure to provide him with everything that he needs to make a correct assessment.

Child Interview

Aside from the parent interview, expect a child interview to take place during an ADHD screening or assessment. Your chosen doctor will most likely want to meet your child personally. Your child may be asked about his understanding of the specific reason for his visit to the doctor. He may also be asked about his perceptions about the specific behavioral concerns and problems that caused the need for an assessment.

The child interview serves as a way to evaluate the developmental skills and behavior of your child in an informal setting. It is because kids tend to behave differently when dealing with an unfamiliar and new one-on-one situation. Medical specialists are aware of that, so when the symptoms that tend to create problems at home and school are not present during the interview, they will immediately take note of that.

Psychological and Educational Tests

Psychological and educational tests also form a huge part of the ADHD screening and assessment. The results of this test are not completely used in diagnosing ADHD, though. However, these could indicate certain concerns about other developmental or emotional issues or learning disabilities. In such a case, expect your doctor to tell you about it.

Physical Examination

Apart from the tests already mentioned, your child might also need to undergo a neurodevelopmental screening and pediatric physical exam. This examination is essential in ruling out other medical problems that might display symptoms similar to ADHD. In some cases, language and formal speech screening and assessment may also be conducted.

Sensory evaluation

During the ADHD screening and evaluation, your sensory functions will be tested. These include your sense of touch, seeing, and hearing. A licensed optometrist or ophthalmologist will be the one to conduct the vision test while an audiologist is required to perform the hearing test. It is important to have the right professionals do these tests because the usual hearing and vision exams conducted in your child's pediatrician's clinic are not that sensitive, causing their inability to identify if there are problems in sensory functions.

As for the sense of touch, you will be the one to evaluate your child first because this one is the most obvious. As you can see, kids who have tactile sensitivity do not usually like extremely cold or hot things. They do not also like it when there are seams in the clothes they wear and if someone brushes their hair. Based on your observation and report, a psychologist will continue evaluating your child's tactile sensitivity. Expect this to be conducted during the part when the psycho-educational assessment is done.

Psycho-educational evaluation

Performed by a licensed psychologist, this vital part of the ADHD screening is a big help in evaluating the emotions, academic functions, cognition, and motor functions of your child. Other professionals can also contribute to this test. These include physical and occupational therapists, social workers, and reading and learning specialists. However, it is the responsibility of the psychologist to collect all important pieces and create the report.

In this specific part of the evaluation, your child's intellectual and cognitive functions will be assessed using a set of tests designed to measure their social judgment, knowledge, abstract thinking, processing speed, memory, visual-spatial functioning, and arithmetic.

The psychologist will also conduct neuropsychological tasks designed to examine the memory, motor function, visual-motor skills, visual-spatial processing, speed of processing, auditory process, and executive functions, including motivation, planning, and organization, of your child.

Furthermore, there is an educational and academic test that will be performed during this stage, assessing whether your child functions based on what is appropriate for his age. Aside from all that, the psychologist will evaluate your child's emotional functions and feelings by examining his responses to various stimuli and situations.

It is crucial to gather all these details even if you, your child, and his teachers already filled up questionnaires regarding his behaviors and development. It is because the gathered info can help point to the right diagnosis.

Auditory Processing Evaluation

Another vital component of the ADHD screening and evaluation process is the auditory processing evaluation. This is an exam, which will be conducted in case your child hears the sound without actually processing what he hears. For instance, your child has problems differentiating various sounds, causing him to mispronounce or mishear a few words. You can also find some kids experiencing difficulty when exposed to noisy environments.

Others, on the other hand, will only respond to a step or two of a request composed of multiple steps. One thing to take note of regarding the problems experienced by your child with speech, reading, and auditory memory is that these might be triggered by difficulties and challenges in auditory processing. This results in your child looking as if he does not remember what you are saying or does not pay attention to.

With the help of the auditory processing evaluation, it is easy to identify whether this problem can be pointed to ADHD. This test is known to be more effective when conducted on kids who are at least 7 years old.

Some Diagnosis Tips

If you want to be able to handle the whole ADHD diagnosis screening process much easier then it is crucial to be guided by a few tips before starting. Some of the tips you have to keep in mind before, during, and after the evaluation are the following:

- Describe the problems in a more specific manner – Before visiting your chosen specialist, make sure that you are already aware of the specific concerns you intend the consultation to be addressed. For instance, you should be specific on the issues and symptoms displayed by your child either at home or school. It could be that he always loses his toys or fails to do his homework.

- Consider your view and stance regarding medications before setting up an appointment – If you are one of those who are opposed to the idea of taking medications then make sure to let the doctor or specialist know about this principle of yours upfront. If that is the case, then you may want to ask for recommendations from the doctor regarding other treatment options.

Also, remember that the intake of medicine is solely up to you. This means that even if the specialist prescribes for your child even if you do not approve of it, you can always decide to look for another doctor. However, if you decided to let your child take medication, keep in mind that the dosing and prescription differ from one individual to another.

This means that you might need to do trial-and-error at first. What you should do is to let your child try different brands and dosages until you figure out the safest and most suitable one for him.

- Discuss various options regarding medications – Make sure that you seek the services of a medical professional who will, aside from writing a prescription, give a detailed discussion of the treatment and diagnosis process. Some of the questions you should raise during the consultation are those regarding the specific medications considered, reasons to begin taking a certain medication, expectations upon taking the medication, and the way the specialist will evaluate the medication's effects.

- Ask about follow-up appointments – It is also advisable to ask the specialist or doctor you have chosen regarding follow-up appointments and treatments. Note that one sign that you are dealing with a good specialist or medical professional for ADHD is when he can give you a more detailed course of action.

The doctor should also be easily accessible. It is because you will most likely need to be in touch with him in the days and weeks that follow the

ADHD screening. This is especially true while you are still trying to figure out the correct and safest dosage for your child.

Among the things that you should consider before choosing a doctor, therefore, are his availability, consultation fees, and the ability to prescribe medication refills via phone. You will also need to know if there is a need for you to visit his office each time your child displays severe symptoms and unwanted behaviors.

- Ask about medication alternatives – Determine if there are alternative behavioral modifications and therapies you can use for your child. Find out if your doctor can do such alternative techniques. It would be a big help if you deal with a doctor who can refer you to a psychologist, someone capable of providing behavioral help when needed. These include dealing with work struggles and some effective time management techniques.

- Find a doctor who is willing to meet your entire family – Note that being diagnosed with ADHD can have a major impact on the lives of people you are living with. This is the main reason why other people who are part of your child's life, especially those who live with him in the household, should also set up an appointment or meeting with the doctor to understand the condition and the basics of managing it.

During the process of evaluating and diagnosing a child with ADHD, the medical specialist or healthcare professional will also provide information about how severe the case is. It is because there are mild, moderate, and severe cases of the disorder. If your child is diagnosed with a mild case of ADHD then expect him to display only minor impairments in the way he functions every day while still showing more than enough symptoms designed to adhere to the criteria and guidelines for diagnosis.

Your child has a moderate case in case the impairment to his daily functioning is more significant than the mild one. Severe cases, on the other hand, display a lot of symptoms. This means that the signs and symptoms displayed by your child are greater in number than what is required minimally for a diagnosis. These symptoms are often accompanied by significant impairments.

How Long Does it Take to Get the Results?

Once all of the tests are conducted, you may be dying to know what the result is. However, avoid expecting to get the answer or result overnight. It is because the ADHD diagnostic process may take at least one or two weeks. With that in mind, make sure that you inform the teachers and other officials in the school in case you are still waiting for the result. Inform them that he is undergoing evaluation for ADHD.

Also, consider setting up a meeting with the special education teacher or psychologist in the school to talk about getting your child assessed and evaluated for learning disorders or disabilities. It is because around thirty to fifty percent of children suffering from ADHD also have learning disabilities.

In case your school can't administer the appropriate tests or exams for some reason, you can always consult a private educational psychologist and have him do it for you. Prepare to spend a few hundred dollars for this, though.

Coping with the Diagnosis of ADHD

It is rare for a parent to start the whole ADHD evaluation and assessment process without worrying about the results. If the outcome is just as what you have suspected, proving that your child indeed has ADHD, then do not lose hope. Note that your parenting forms a vital part of treating the condition.

This is why you should try to give as much help as you can. Also, remember that your response to the result of the evaluation can make coping with ADHD either easy or hard. However, now that you received the diagnosis, your first concern would be where and how you should begin when it comes to helping your child cope.

Learning about the actual diagnosis is helpful but fully understanding what it specifically means not only for your child but also for you and the entire family can help in setting up the right support system. Here are some of the steps that you should take to make the process of coping much easier after the diagnosis:

Discuss the diagnosis with your child

Of course, this should be the first step that you have to take after the diagnosis. Explain the result to him. As a parent of an ADHD child, you have to teach him about his condition, including its effects on his relationship with friends and school experiences. This is not meant to frighten your child.

Wide knowledge of his condition can empower him. It can make him fully understand what he is going through and how he can manage his symptoms. While this discussion can be difficult and challenging at first, especially if your child is still too young, you can rest assured that with proper talking points, you can handle the discussion well.

One way to do it is to give him a talk about the human brain. Tell him that each person has his style of learning. Each one is unique, too. It is because you can't find two brains that are the same. This is why his brain seems to work too fast, making it difficult for him to process his thoughts, wait for a while before he starts talking, or sit still.

Tell him that while having a brain that works too fast is one of his strengths, this might also be problematic at times so you should work together to manage it, especially during tough times. Also, empower him that many successful people suffer from ADHD. Let him know that this condition is not something to be frightened of or embarrassed about.

Check the web to find famous leaders and people who have ADHD so your child will feel empowered upon seeing them as role models. It is also advisable to be realistic about the condition. This means that you have to tell him the truth that ADHD is not something that both of you can treat overnight.

However, you can work together to implement some techniques that will decrease those components of ADHD that make him feel stressed, including trouble with friends, being called out in class, and certain outbursts. As much as possible, discuss your coping or treatment plan with him. Inform him about the medications he can take and the coping strategies you can apply both at home and in school.

Talking about medications, make sure that you discuss this with your child without sounding negative. Let him know the importance of medication in managing ADHD symptoms that he might be unable to control. You should also teach your child the importance of doing regular physical activities, especially in reducing severe symptoms of ADHD and improving cognitive function.

By letting your child know the importance of doing extra exercises and letting him know more about movement techniques that are applicable in the classroom, he will have a higher chance of coping. It lets him know the basics of helping himself, allowing him to take control of his situation.

Study-related emotional and behavioral issues

Another step that you should take during the coping period is to gather as much information as you can about various emotional and behavioral issues. Keep in mind that one common complication of ADHD in children is that it also tends to cause the development of other mental health issues.

It is quick to diagnose children who have behavioral issues and are highly disruptive. However, they are also among those who seem to struggle to maintain and make friends, deal with classroom consequences, and build poor self-esteem the most. ADHD kids who are inattentive may not deal with a lot of behavioral interruptions but are at risk of having a difficult time maintaining their focus. This effect can have a significant impact on their performance at school and their learning development.

Also, take note that thirty percent of those who were diagnosed with ADHD during their childhood years carried the condition upon reaching adulthood. Those who were diagnosed with the condition during childhood are also prone to suffering from an antisocial personality disorder, substance abuse, depression, and anxiety. Some of them even have suicidal thoughts.

With that in mind, it is crucial to learn about these emotional and behavioral issues together with gathering as much info as you can about ADHD. It is because these issues are related to your child's diagnosed condition. By knowing about such related conditions, you can find the appropriate support whenever needed.

Also, take note that there are some ADHD signs and symptoms that tend to mask other issues and problems. Learn about these so an accurate evaluation and diagnosis will be given, allowing you to find the most appropriate treatment and action plan for your child.

Study treatment options

Another essential step is to study various treatment options for kids who suffer from ADHD. Note that while ADHD treatment is complex, especially for children, it is still possible to find the most suitable approach if parents, teachers, school officials, psychologists, and healthcare professionals work together.

A team approach ensures that the child has supported both in the home and in the school setting. If you want to have a more detailed plan then it helps if you follow these steps:

- Look for a neuropsychologist who can evaluate your child even more - Set up a meeting with your chosen neuropsychologist. The goal here is to review, evaluate, and comprehend the testing results. It is also advisable to talk about the specific behavioral strategies and accommodations that are beneficial for your child both at home and school.

- Show the test results when seeking medication evaluation – Make sure that the test results are with you when you are meeting your medical doctor to get a medication evaluation. It is also advisable to sign releases that will allow all parties involved to work together. Your goal is to work as a team so your child can get as much support as he needs. Make sure that his classroom teacher is also part of the team.

- Find a cognitive behavioral therapist – This is a big help when trying to correct some of your child's unwanted and impulsive behaviors. If you have no idea about a therapist whom you can work with, then you can always ask for referrals from your neuropsychologist.

- Talk to other parents – If possible, talk with parents who also have children suffering from ADHD. This is a huge help in trading coping and recovering advice and tips and seeking the support needed while navigating the recovery process.

- Ask for a team meeting that will be held at school – Make sure that all members of your support team are present during the meeting. These include your cognitive-behavioral therapist, neuropsychologist, and other professionals who work with you to give the support plan needed by your child.

Talk to the school about your chosen treatment plan

Once you have created a treatment plan for your child, make sure to discuss this with the school. Set up an appointment with the school support services and classroom teacher. Your goal is to have a scheduled meeting with them, so you can discuss the informal supports and the class accommodations that your child should get at school.

It could be providing tools to lessen his tendency to fidget or letting him sit close to the class teacher. You may also discuss other coping techniques, like giving extensions during tests and when giving assignments and using graphs and pictures that can help your child learn more.

Making the Coping or Treatment Plan Work

While it can be overwhelming and frustrating the moment you confirm that your child indeed has ADHD through the diagnosis of a medical professional, you can still eliminate all your worries and frustrations once you realize that you have a supportive team and a good treatment plan in place. You can make the coping plan work in your favor with the right support and all the vital school and home interventions set up.

Also, do not lose hope if your child is diagnosed with ADHD. The diagnosis will even serve as a good wake-up call. It is even designed to provide you the additional push needed to start seeking help designed to lessen the symptoms experienced by your child, especially those that tend to affect his success and happiness.

After confirming the presence of the condition, make sure that you act on it fast. Avoid waiting for too long to begin treatment. Note that the earlier you start dealing with the symptoms, the better it will be for you and your child. To make the treatment plan work, keep in mind that managing the symptoms of the condition takes a lot of hard work.

Also, figuring out the most suitable treatment requires trial and error and a generous dose of persistence and time. Still, you can make everything work in your child's favor – that is by reminding yourself about your goals. It is also advisable to incorporate the following key principles in the treatment plan – strong knowledge about ADHD, healthy lifestyle habits, and adequate support.

Chapter 3 – Managing Life with ADHD

Now that your child is diagnosed with ADHD, it is time to take the necessary steps to raise him into a successful person despite having the disorder. True, raising an ADHD-afflicted child is not the same as the traditional approach to child-rearing. It is because normal household routines and rule-making will be impossible to set up. It is also advisable to implement an approach based on the severity and type of symptoms experienced by your child.

To help you in guiding your child to take full control over his life despite having ADHD, you, as the parent, should accept him and his condition wholeheartedly. Accept the fact that those who suffer from this condition have brains that are functionally different when compared to other kids.

Another thing to remember is that while kids suffering from ADHD are still capable of learning acceptable and non-acceptable behaviors, the disorder may still cause them to become impulsive. You may feel frustrated with all the behaviors that your child displays because of his ADHD but you can rest assured that there are certain techniques designed to make his life easier to manage.

Also, remember that nurturing your child's development with the condition means modifying some of your behaviors and finding ways to manage your child's behaviors. It would be best to start the treatment at home because this is where your child will receive all the genuine love and support that he specifically needs.

Make sure that everyone in the household is aware of his condition, too. This way, everyone will be able to serve as a strong means of support for him. As a parent, your goal should be to help him overcome daily struggles and challenges, inject calmness into the family and channel his excessive energy into something positive.

The more consistent and quicker you are in addressing his struggles and problems, the higher your chance of helping him succeed in life despite his disorder. Also, remember that while you are frustrated with your child's condition, the whole journey will also be as frustrating and overwhelming for him as what you feel.

By keeping that in mind, it will be easier for you to respond in ways that are positive for him and make him feel your support. It is also necessary to start building a happy and stable home for him – one that can help him manage and deal with the childhood symptoms of ADHD because of the support, love, patience, and compassion of the people around him.

Making the Entire Family Understand

To succeed in parenting a child who is suffering from ADHD, it is necessary to learn about how his symptoms will affect the whole family. Note that ADHD-afflicted kids are prone to exhibit a set of behaviors and symptoms capable of disrupting family life. For instance, you can't expect them to obey all the time because they frequently do not hear instructions from their parents. They are also easily distracted and disorganized, causing other members of the family to wait. There are also instances when ADHD kids begin tasks and projects only to forget finishing and cleaning them up.

Those who are prone to displaying impulsive behaviors are at risk of demanding attention during inappropriate times, interrupting conversations, saying embarrassing and insensitive things, and speaking before thinking. Parents of kids with ADHD might also have a hard time putting their children to sleep. For extremely hyperactive kids, they may not only mess up the household but also put themselves at risk.

Due to the destructive and impulsive behaviors of a child with ADHD, everyone in the family, including siblings and other relatives living with him may struggle at first. If you have other children then expect them to receive less attention compared to your child suffering from ADHD. You may rebuke others more sharply in case they complain about something or do something bad. There is also a high chance that you will take their successes for granted or celebrate them less.

For siblings who are tasked to act as assistant parents when both you and your spouse are not around, they are at risk of getting blamed in case the one with ADHD displays unwanted behaviors that put him in danger under their supervision. Eventually, this might cause them to resent or envy your child with ADHD.

With all these effects of parenting a child diagnosed with ADHD, it is safe to assume that the demands involved in monitoring and taking care of him can be mentally draining and physically exhausting. The fact that he can't listen to you intently might result in frustration that will eventually lead to anger. The problem is that you will also feel guilty for feeling that way once your anger subsides.

The whole rollercoaster of emotions can cause you to feel stressed and anxious. This is why you have to nurture a home where everyone truly understands the situation of your child. Make his siblings learn about his condition, too, so they will be able to accept him wholeheartedly without resenting him in the long run. Both you and your partner, together with your children and the entire family, should build a home with consistency and compassion.

If possible, make everyone meet up with your child's doctor or specialist so they will better understand what your child is going through. Your goal is to create a home that provides your child with the structure and love he needs to manage his symptoms.

To nurture such a home, the following guidelines and tips can help. All these are designed to limit your child's destructive and impulsive behaviors while also overcoming his self-doubts:

Remain positive

Being the parent, you are the one who is responsible for setting up the stage of your child's physical and emotional health. It is you who have full control over several factors that can influence his symptoms positively. With that in mind, it is crucial to show and maintain your positivity all the time. This is the key to guiding your child in dealing with his struggles and challenges.

By staying focused and calm, you increase your chance of connecting to your child, making him as focused and calm as possible, too. Hold your judgment and remain calm when your child displays unwanted and embarrassing behaviors. Remember that such behaviors are only the results of a disorder. They are not intentional, so avoid resenting or scolding your child because of these.

Be willing to compromise, too. Show how positive you are by not minding the small stuff too much. For instance, if your child was unable to finish one task, avoid making a huge deal out of it, especially if he was able to complete a couple of tasks successfully. Avoid being a perfectionist as this might only lead to dissatisfaction. Furthermore, this might cause you to set high and impossible expectations from your ADHD-afflicted child.

Another thing that you can do to retain a positive attitude is to continue believing in your child and his abilities. Have faith in him. What you can do is to list down all the things that are unique, valuable, and positive about him. Believe in his ability to mature, succeed, change, and learn. Reaffirm your faith and trust in him every day.

Take good care of yourself and your health

Remember that you are the ultimate source of strength and the role model of your child. With that in mind, you need to try living a healthy and happy life. If you do not take good care of yourself and your health then you will be at risk of being overly exhausted, causing you to run out of patience often. If that happens, then you will also be at risk of destroying the support and structure you have built for him.

One of the things that you can do for yourself is to ask for support. Remember that you do not have to be alone in raising your child. You can always get the support and help of others, like your child's teachers, therapist, and doctor. You can also get rid of some of the piled-up burdens from your chest by participating in support groups composed of parents of ADHD-afflicted kids.

The good thing about being a part of this support group is that you gain access to a forum that lets you give and receive advice. It is also one of the safest places where you can share your experiences and vent out your pent-up emotions and feelings. Do not forget to take a break, too.

Do not feel guilty each time you ask the help of trusted friends and family to babysit your child. Note that you also need time to breathe and focus on yourself. Accept any offer of help but make sure to talk to them honestly about how they can effectively handle and manage the symptoms of your child.

Do not neglect your health, too. Nurture yourself and improve your health by eating right, exercising, and looking for ways to lessen stress. It could be meditating every morning or taking a warm bath every night. Also, make sure to recognize it in case you get sick. Ask for help if necessary.

Build structure and set routines at home

Ensure that everyone follows the structure and routines you have established. Note that most of those who have ADHD have a higher chance of succeeding in task completion if they are required to fulfill their tasks and activities in predictable places and patterns. This is why building a structure at home and sustaining it is important. This will allow your child to understand what to expect from the people in the household and what others expect him to do, as well.

To build a more structured home with routines that will help improve the focus and organizational skills of your child, apply the following tips:

- **Create predictable routines** – Set a place and schedule for everything that your child needs to do so he can meet and fully understand expectations. For example, you can build predictable and simple rituals for bedtime, play, homework, and meals.

  You may also want to train your child to prepare the clothes he will wear the next day before he sleeps. Also, look for a special and easily accessible spot where you can put all the things that he needs for school. That way, you can prepare everything, ready for him to grab anytime.

- **Surround your home with timers and clocks** – Ensure that your home is filled with clocks and timers. Put a huge one in his bedroom, too. This will allow him to understand the value of doing things on schedule. Just make sure that you also give him sufficient time to finish his tasks, such as when he is preparing what he needs to bring to school or when doing his homework. A timer also needs to be used for transitional times or homework (ex. between playtime and preparing for bed).

- **Keep his schedule simple** – When creating a schedule for your child, make it as simple as possible. Also, remember that while it is beneficial to ensure that he does not have any idle time in his schedule, he will become more prone to distractions and get wound up if you fill his day with too many activities after school.

  With that in mind, be prepared to adjust his schedule and commitments after school depending on his skills and abilities. Consider the demands of a specific activity, too. Do not give him too much idle time as this might only aggravate his symptoms and cause chaos at home. However, try to make his activities as simple as possible. Avoid piling on too many complex tasks and activities as such might only overwhelm him.

- **Set aside a quiet spot for him** – Another way to build a home that can nurture your child with ADHD is to set aside a quiet spot for him. This should be his private space. It could be a bedroom or a part of your porch. You should set this private spot for him to organize his thoughts and calm his overactive behaviors.

- **Keep your home as neat and organized as possible** – Do everything you can to organize your home and avoid mess as much as possible. Your goal is to make sure your child understands how important it is to put everything in the right places. Show him the importance of being organized and neat by leading by example.

- **Keep him busy** – You may want to sign him up for music and art classes, and sports. You can also keep him busy while at home by organizing simple activities designed to fill up his time. Among the simple tasks and activities that you can ask him to do are drawing pictures, playing board games with his sibling, and assisting you when cooking.

  Avoid relying too much on video and computer games and TV shows when trying to occupy his time. It is because some video games and TV shows are naturally violent, thereby aggravating your child's ADHD symptoms.

All these tips can help you build a more predictable and productive day for your child. By setting up routines, your home will become a more structured place for him, allowing him to move following what is right eventually.

Encourage him to move

Note that kids with ADHD usually have a lot of spare energy. Because of that, you need to focus on encouraging him to move. You can organize physical activities for him, like letting him play his favorite sports, so you can drain his energy through healthy means. The good thing about stimulating movement is that it also allows him to focus his attention on specific skills and movements.

Physical activities also have endless benefits for him – among which are reduced risk of suffering from anxiety and depression, better brain development and growth, and improved focus and concentration. Furthermore, the fact that he moves and exercises a lot also promotes a better quality of sleep. This is a good thing when planning to reduce his symptoms.

When choosing an activity for him, make sure to go for one that he will surely enjoy. It should also be a sport or activity that perfectly suits his strengths. Softball and other sports that have plenty of downtimes, for instance, are not suitable for your child if his symptoms usually point to problems in attention and focus. In such a case, it would be better to get him involved in a team and individual sports, such as hockey and basketball, as these require them to move constantly.

Young ADHD sufferers will also find it beneficial to undergo martial arts training as tae kwon do. They can also practice yoga. It is because both martial arts and yoga are effective in boosting mental control while giving the body sufficient workout.

Ensure that he gets enough sleep

Another way to help your child manage ADHD symptoms at home is to ensure that he gets sufficient sleep every night. Everyone knows how poor and insufficient sleep can greatly affect one's focus and attention. The problem is that its impact is even more detrimental to kids suffering from ADHD.

Being diagnosed with ADHD, your child requires the same amount of sleep as other kids without the problem. However, he usually does not get what he needs. It is because problems regarding focus and attention might overstimulate his mind, causing difficulties when trying to fall asleep.

If you want him to get enough sleep and beat such a problem then it would be helpful to set an early bedtime schedule for him. Make sure to be consistent in making him follow that routine. Among the things that you can do to encourage your child to get sufficient rest and sleep are:

- Reducing screen and television time

- Increasing the levels of exercise and physical activities throughout the day

- Getting rid of caffeine from his daily diet

- Cuddling for at least 10 minutes – This is a great way to make him feel your love. With that, he will calm down knowing that he is secure with you by his side.

- Putting some calming aromas, like lavender in his room – The relaxing scent is usually enough to calm a hyperactive child.

- Lessening his level of physical activity around one hour before his bedtime schedule – You may still occupy his time during this period, but make sure to choose quieter and calmer activities, like quiet play, reading, and coloring books.

- Play relaxing background noise – You may play some relaxation tapes so there will be a soothing background noise when he is trying to fall asleep. The good news is that you can choose from a wide range of sounds, including calming music and those that come from nature. You may also play white noise in the background. It is even possible for you to make white noise yourself – that is by letting an electric fan run or setting a radio on static.

Set rules at home

Coping with ADHD symptoms will also be easier at home if you establish clear rules and expectations and let your child know about them. Explain the rules and expectations clearly. One thing you have to take note of about kids with ADHD is that they need rules and guidelines that they can consistently follow and understand. As for your own home, make sure that you set behavioral rules and guidelines that are clear and easy to understand.

To increase the chance of your child following the rules and not forgetting them, it would be best to write them down. You should then hang the list in a spot where he can see and read the rules easily. When setting rules at home, it is also important to remind yourself that kids diagnosed with ADHD tend to deliver appropriate responses if you expose them to well-organized systems composed of consequences and rewards.

Let them know the consequences if they violate the rules. Stick to the system you have set, too. Make sure to follow the rules. However, you should not only focus on the consequences. You also have to set up some rewards that your child will surely enjoy if he was able to stick to the system.

Remember that when establishing consistent structures, your child will also most likely receive criticisms frequently. Because of that, you should also try to work on giving him rewards every time he shows good behavior. Observe him closely and give him praises each time he does something right. Rewards and praises are especially vital for kids diagnosed with ADHD since they only receive a bit of these.

Most of them only receive complaints, remediation, criticisms, and corrections because of their behavior. They only gain a bit of positive reinforcement so try to be as generous as possible with rewards and praises to encourage your child to try showing only good behaviors. Fortunately, you do not have to splurge when it comes to rewards.

Simple praise, positive comment, or a smile can already boost his concentration and attention. It can also motivate him to try controlling his impulsive behaviors. While it can be difficult at times, try to focus more on sending him positive praise for completing tasks and displaying appropriate behaviors and providing only little negative responses and criticisms for poor performance and inappropriate behaviors.

Give him rewards for even minor achievements and progress that you will most likely ignore from another normal child. When it comes to rewards, it would be best to:

- Give him praises, positive activities, and privileges instead of toys and foods

- Adjust or make changes on the rewards often – It is because his condition might cause him to get bored with the reward if you do not change it a bit.

- Create a chart that shows the stars and points you awarded him each time he displays good behaviors – This will serve as his visual reminder that there are also times when he succeeded in controlling his unwanted behavior.

In terms of consequences, make sure that you explain them in detail to your child in advance. You have to make them know what to expect in case they misbehaved. In the case of misbehaviors, among the most viable consequences that you can use are time-outs and removing certain privileges.

It also helps to observe your child so you will know what triggers him to misbehave. By doing that, you can immediately take him out of environments and situations that serve as triggers for some of his inappropriate behaviors.

Encourage him to develop healthy eating habits

Parenting your child who has ADHD at home also requires you to guide him when it comes to eating right. Note that while your child's diet does not cause the disorder directly, you still have to remember that the foods he takes in can have a major impact on his mental state. This will also affect his behavior. This is why you have to do something to modify and monitor how much, when, and what he eats. By doing that, you can sort of lessen the symptoms he is displaying.

All kids, not just those suffering from ADHD, can gain a lot of benefits from regular healthy meal times and fresh foods. It is also beneficial for them to avoid junk and processed foods. This is the reason why these should serve as your guiding principles when creating a healthy diet plan for your child. Keep in mind that his distractedness and impulsiveness might cause overeating, disordered eating, and missed meals, so you have to focus on making him establish healthy eating habits.

Also, kids diagnosed with ADHD are prone to not eating regular meals. Without proper guidance from parents or guardians, they will be at risk of not eating for several hours then binging on whatever food laid out in front of them. This unhealthy pattern can lead to devastating effects on their emotional and physical health.

To ensure that this will not happen to your child, make sure to do something to prevent him from developing unhealthy and unwanted eating habits. Ensure that he does not develop unhealthy and poor eating habits by setting a regular schedule for him to eat nutritious snacks or meals. If possible, his meals or snacks should not go over three hours apart.

To improve his physical health, you need to let him take healthy foods regularly. Eating on schedule is also good for him mentally, knowing that these serve as a way for him to take a break from a busy day. To ensure that your ADHD-diagnosed child is eating right, eliminate junk foods from your home. If you need to eat out, ensure that sugary and fatty foods are inaccessible to him.

Another way to prevent your child from developing unhealthy eating habits is to turn off any TV show that is filled with a lot of ads for junk and processed foods. Do not forget to pair up his healthy mealtimes with vitamin and mineral supplements, too.

Break down tasks, especially complex ones, into easy-to-manage chunks

Note that due to ADHD, your child may find some tasks and activities at home too off-putting and complicated. This is the main reason why you have to look for a way to break down tasks into chunks that they can easily manage and achieve. This is a great way to simplify their tasks at home while controlling and regulating their emotions, especially those linked to failures and success.

For instance, if you ask your child to clean his room, it helps to break down this one task into smaller ones to prevent him from getting too overwhelmed. Some sub-tasks that you can create out of this include make the bed, fold clothes, and return toys to their proper storage places.

You may also find a large wall calendar helpful in reminding your child of the tasks and duties at hand. Put this calendar in a specific spot in your home where he can easily see. Another tip is to apply the color-coding scheme for homework and household chores. This scheme is a big help in preventing your child from getting too overwhelmed with his school assignments and daily tasks. It also helps to break down even his regular morning routines into smaller and more discreet ones.

Other Do's and Don'ts when Parenting a Child with ADHD at Home

To make the process of parenting your child with ADHD easier to do at home, make sure that you also follow these simple do's and don'ts:

- **Limit distractions** – A child diagnosed with ADHD will have a much simpler life if you keep possible distractions to a minimum. Remember that because of the disorder, your child is prone to welcoming distractions that he can easily access. These include video games, television, and computer that might only stimulate impulsive and inappropriate behaviors. Due to that possibility, make sure to regulate his exposure to the mentioned distractions.

  Try to reduce the amount of time he spends on electronics, gadgets, and the screen. What you should do, instead, is to let him spend more time engaging in outdoor activities. This is a good way to have an effective outlet for all his excess energy. It also helps to organize and simplify the life of your child.

If possible, build a quiet and special space for him where he can do his homework, read, or do other activities he loves without distractions. This spot should also serve as his outlet for taking a break from his somewhat chaotic daily life.

Also, your home should be kept as neat and as organized as possible. Let him know where certain items at home should go. By doing that, you can lessen, if not fully eliminate, unnecessary and unwanted distractions.

- **Encourage him to think aloud** – The fact that your child has ADHD may cause him to lack self-control, causing him to act and speak before thinking. This is also the main reason why you should train him to think aloud at home. Allow him to verbalize his reasoning and thoughts each time he feels the urge to misbehave or act out.

As a parent, you have to gain a full understanding of the thought process of your child. This is the key to helping him curb and fight impulsive and unwanted behaviors. Teach him the concept of wait time, too. This involves pausing for a moment before he responds to a situation or talks.

The good thing about the wait time concept is that it allows him to have full control of his impulse and urge to speak and behave without thinking it through first. Another tip is to train him on how to respond thoughtfully. You can do that by helping him with his assignments or by asking him interactive questions regarding his favorite book or TV show.

- **Prioritize his safety** – Make sure that your home serves as the safest place for him. Pay attention to his safety once he is at home. Note that due to ADHD, your child may be unaware of the dangers surrounding him. This can make him prone to getting hurt. This is the main reason why you have to get rid of anything in your home that might put him in danger. These include firearms, tools, like lawnmowers, and poisonous chemicals, medicines, and cleaning supplies.

Prioritize the safety of your child when it comes to taking his medicines, too. This means that if his doctor prescribes a medicine that he needs to take at a designated time and recommended dose then make sure to stick with it. Do not give medicines at a dosage that is not recommended. Ensure that the medicines are stored in a safe place at home, too.

- **Give yourself a break** – Remember that you will be unable to give your 100 percent support to your child if you feel exhausted and stressed. Give yourself a break from time to time so you can breathe. Also, do not feel bad if you get frustrated or overwhelmed not only with the situation but also with your child and yourself. It is normal to feel that way.

What you should do if that happens is to breathe and relax. Just like your child, you also need to have a break. As a parent, it is also helpful to have your own alone time. You can always hire a babysitter or ask for the help of your trusted friends or relatives to take care of your child during your scheduled alone time.

Just make sure that you explain to them the things that they should and should not do to manage your child's behaviors. During your alone time, do things that can relieve your stress, including working out in a gym, taking a walk, enjoying a warm and relaxing bath, and meditating.

- **Learn ways to calm yourself** – It would be impossible for you to offer your help to your impulsive and hyperactive child if you are also aggravated and stressed. Children, especially those with ADHD, are also prone to mimicking the behaviors of people surrounding them. With that in mind, try to be as calm as possible, even during outbursts.

  Practice ways to stay controlled and composed even during those times when your child misbehaves. This will allow him to do the same, too. Spend a few minutes to breathe, collect your thoughts, and relax before trying to soothe or pacify him. If you feel calm when dealing with him, then you can also expect him to calm down.

- **Discipline with warmth, love, and purpose** – Find out what specific approaches will help you discipline your child more effectively. Determine those methods that might worsen ADHD symptoms. Your goal is to discipline him at home in a way that he will feel your love and warmth and understand the purpose.

If possible, gain coaching from the therapist of your child so you can find means to respond better to his behavior. Also, remember that most children suffering from the disorder are sensitive to criticisms. With that in mind, try to correct your child's behavior in a supportive and encouraging manner. Do not make it punishing.

- **Spend special moments together** – Ensure that you spend some special time with your child every day. Bond with him. You should be able to set aside some time every day to talk to him and do fun, exciting, and relaxing activities with him. Even just a few minutes of your day will work wonders.

During this time, ensure that he receives your full attention. If he displays positive and appropriate behaviors, do not forget to give compliments. Avoid overpraising, though. The goal is to just let him know that he did something good. If you noticed that he is waiting patiently for his turn, for instance, then tell him that what he did is great.

- **Do not command; instead, explain** – As a parent, you can always provide age-appropriate reasons every time you ask your child to do something. Find simple reasons and explain them to your child elaborately. Instead of commanding your child to do a specific task, give him reasons why he needs to do it. This helps alleviate his confusion and worries.

  Every time you try to explain the reason for a task, it is important to utilize clear and positive language. Your attempt to explain everything to your child is also a great way to show how much you respect him, which can make him feel good, especially if he starts to feel that he is different from the others.

- **Do not use negative language** – When taking care of your child with ADHD at home, avoid using negative language as much as possible. Learn to provide positive feedback as much as possible, which is the key to building his confidence. Note that because of your child's disorder, there are times when he feels like people dislike him or that everything he does is wrong.

Do not reinforce such thoughts by using negative language at home. Doing so might only hurt him and worsen his disruptive behaviors. However, you may struggle to stay positive at all times. This is the reason why you have to take the tips on calming yourself and learning to relax seriously.

Look for outlets where you can express all your worries and concerns. This could be your partner, friend, family member, or therapist. You can also find groups online composed of members who have the same problems as you. By talking to them, you can release your frustrations while also learning from them.

- **Do not teach your child a lot of things all at once** – It would be best to focus on making him learn one task at a time. Avoid filling his head with too much knowledge and tasks all at once. Begin small and choose one task that you want him to concentrate on. Do not forget to give your child praise for his effort to learn.

Parenting an ADHD-diagnosed child can be hard and frustrating at first but you will be able to get the hang of it soon. Nurture a loving home for him, so he will love the idea of family. Note that your relationship with him is what matters the most right now. He may always feel like he is letting other people down, he is not good at anything, or he always does things incorrectly.

Try to protect his self-esteem by building a home filled with people who can understand and accept him. Be patient and make him realize how much you believe in him. Also, let him know that you see a lot of positive traits from him. Establish resilience by building a loving and positive relationship with your child and giving him a home where he can feel safe and fully protected.

Managing your Child's ADHD at School

Another aspect of your child's life that you have to focus on after he gets diagnosed with ADHD is his academics. Note that school is challenging for kids dealing with ADHD. Despite that, there are still ways for you to help your child succeed and learn something in class. One of the things that you should do first is to set up a meeting with his teachers. You have to talk to them so you can relay the goals and needs of your child.

The meeting should also serve as a way for you to determine how his teachers can help him while he is in the classroom. Among the things that his teachers can do is to let him sit in front and ensure that he is not close to the windows and doors. It is a good spot for him as it can prevent him from distractions, thereby helping him remain focused.

Being in the front row will also let his teacher see whether your child needs a bit of help. It also helps to create a daily schedule for your child as well as a behavioral plan in written form that encourages him to do positive acts. Post this schedule and plan on your child's desk or a wall close to him. That way, he can see it all the time.

Another thing that you have to constantly remind yourself of is that your child will find the classroom environment constantly challenging because the daily tasks where they have trouble, particularly staying focused, listening intently, and sitting still, are also the specific tasks that they have to do the whole time they are at school.

The most challenging and frustrating out of all these is that he might be among the majority of ADHD-afflicted children who have a strong drive to learn and act in the same way as their peers who do not have the disorder. The problem is that it is not the unwillingness of your child that causes him to learn through traditional means. It is his neurological deficit.

It should also be noted that most of the symptoms of ADHD hurt his ability to gain access to the classroom curriculum. He might also be dealing with a few challenges while inside the school premises and classroom. Among these challenges are:

- Problems sitting still
- Lack of focus during classrooms and when handling worksheets
- Distractions, including other kids, windows, and interesting graphics and posters on walls
- Poor organizational skills, causing him to misplace important folders and papers and forget assignments
- Talking excessively
- Poor motor skills, causing problems in writing assignments and taking notes
- Struggles in accomplishing long-term projects on his own

- Difficulty following directions and instructions

Due to ADHD, your child will also be prone to repetitive negative interactions not only with other kids but also with teachers. His symptoms might also trigger him to develop low self-esteem and make him vulnerable to bullying, teasing, and poor academic performance. This is where your role as a parent becomes important. What you should do is to be your child's support and guide in coping with the deficits and overcoming the challenges and struggles created by the school.

The best way to handle the challenges is to work together with your child in implementing practical solutions and strategies to let him learn not only inside the school but also outside. Communicate with his teachers, too, so you will get an idea about the best learning method for him. Give him the support he needs consistently.

Ask if certain school accommodations can help ADHD-afflicted students, like your child. However, you have to figure out the specific needs of your child in the classroom first. In that case, his teacher and other support staff in the school can help. Once you have determined his needs, it will be easier to determine the specific accommodations that you might want to ask from the school.

Among the accommodations that your child will surely find valuable inside the classroom are:

- Written and oral instructions – It would be a big help if his teachers will try to reiterate oral instructions and write them down for your child.

- Preferential seating – If possible, his seat should be close to the teacher and in front. It should not be close to the windows and any other source of distraction for him.

- Highlighted key points – If there are essential words in the instructions on tests and worksheets, it would be much better if these are highlighted. Highlighted keywords are extremely helpful in making your child focus.

- Breakdown of tasks and assignments – Another accommodation that will surely be of help to your child is the breakdown of huge tasks and assignments into smaller and more manageable pieces. For example, for long assignments, teachers should try to break them down (ex. 5 math problems then followed by another 5 until your child completes it). However, there should be a deadline for each piece to ensure that your child will target it.

- Assistive technology – The school should also try to make your child use assistive technology to learn in the classroom. It is a big help in making the whole learning process more interesting and visual for him.

- Extended deadline during tests – During exams, your ADHD-afflicted child will be able to thrive if timed tests are eliminated. Extended deadlines should also be provided.

- Supervised organization – Another accommodation that the school may be able to provide to your child with ADHD is supervised organization. It could be in the form of a daily backpack and desk cleanup with proper supervision every day. This will train your child to learn more about the proper organization. Your child can also benefit from using color-coded folders and a homework planner, which his teacher should check every day.

- Checklists – If possible, request a detailed checklist of study and organization skills, assignments, and mistakes that your child frequently displays. This list is a big help in letting him stay on track when doing a task while also avoiding mistakes repeatedly.

Aside from requesting special accommodations and supervision, you should also implement the following techniques and strategies designed to help him enjoy the learning process, overcome educational and learning challenges, and experience academic success:

Work together with your child's teacher

Before seeking the help of his teacher, though, remember that this teaching professional already has a lot on his plate. Aside from having to manage a group of kids who have different learning styles and personalities, it is also highly likely that the classroom has a student suffering from ADHD. Because of the many things that the teacher also does every day, avoid relying too much on him.

You can rest assured, though, that his teachers will do their best to assist and help your ADHD-diagnosed child. However, keep in mind that your strong parental involvement is still the key to boosting his education. You are the one who has the strongest power to optimize the chances of your child to achieve success. All it takes is to give him the support he needs when taking a few steps to learn in the classroom.

You can achieve much better and more desirable results if you gain some help and support from his teacher. By working with teachers, parents of ADHD-afflicted kids, like you, can give their children the best experience at school. Fortunately, there are several ways for you to work together with teaching professionals to ensure that your child gets on track while trying to learn at school.

For instance, both parties can work together to guide your child in learning the ins and outs of the classroom and how to handle the struggles and challenges of their day at school. Make sure that you also act as the advocate and voice of your child. You can do so by communicating his needs to the teaching professionals who are directly involved in his learning experience. Just make sure that you also listen to the things that the school officials and teachers have to say.

Listen to their observations and be open to constructive criticisms. You should have a mutual purpose of figuring out the best way to guide your child to succeed. When talking to your child's teachers, whether personally or via email or phone, make sure that you are specific, calm, and positive. Showing a positive attitude while dealing with teachers and school officials can assure you of being able to communicate the needs of your child more effectively.

The following tips can also help you work hand in hand with the teachers of the school and its officials in helping your child attain success in the field of learning:

- **Plan in advance** – It would be much better for you to set or arrange an appointment with the school's teachers and officials before the beginning of the school year. This is beneficial if you want your child to start fresh and with a clean slate. If in case the school year already began, consider talking to the school's counselor or teacher at least once every month.

- **Arrange for meetings** – Set an appointment with the teacher. Make sure that the scheduled meeting is based on a time that is acceptable and favorable for both parties. Stick to the scheduled meeting, too.

Ask his teacher if it would not be an inconvenience to set the meeting in the actual classroom your child is in. If he agrees then grab this opportunity to have a closer look and sense of the actual physical learning environment of your child.

- **Set goals** – Make sure that the goals are created by both parties – you and your partner, as the parents, and the teacher. To set the goals, talk about what you are hoping for your child to experience in school. Determine how you want him to succeed while in school. Together with his teacher, create a list of realistic and specific goals. Discuss certain techniques and methods that can help your child achieve them.

- **Be a good listener** – Listen intently to what his teacher wants to say. Note that just like you, the teacher also wishes your child to become successful in school. Focus on the message of the teacher, even if he is talking about the negative things he observed about your child.

No matter how hard it is to learn about some negative observations, it is still the key to understanding what your child is going through at school. It can help you get to know more about his struggles at school, allowing you to find more effective solutions.

- **Do not hesitate to share some relevant information about your child** – Since you are fully aware of your own child's history, you can relay this info to his teacher. Also, the teacher gets to see him daily, so he can provide you with details about your child that you have to know.

  Together, you can share a lot of details designed to help you gain a much better understanding of the struggles and hardships experienced by your child at school. Make it a point to share observations and information freely and without hesitation. This will encourage his teacher to follow your lead.

- **Ask questions, no matter how hard you think they are** – Do not hesitate to raise some difficult questions during the scheduled meeting with the teacher. One question that you might want to ask is whether or not your child has a specific attitude and behavioral problems while in school, including the playground.

Also, ask whether your child is qualified or eligible to take advantage of special services designed to help him learn academically. Apart from asking questions, do not forget to give the teacher a clear and complete picture of what is happening to your child.

It even helps to give him a list of all the medications that your child has to take. Discuss to him some other treatments that your child is taking. Also, let the teacher know the specific tactics that work as well as those that don't when you implement them at home. His teacher might be able to apply the same tactics when your child suddenly misbehaves in school.

Create and implement a behavior plan

Kids suffering from ADHD can display appropriate behaviors in class. However, they need to have clear expectations and structures so they can also monitor and keep track of their signs and symptoms. If you want to be of help to your child in lessening his symptoms in school then consider creating a behavior plan for him. Make sure to stick to whatever it is that is stated in the plan.

Also, regardless of the kind of behavior plan, you intend to create and implement, make sure to develop it while closely collaborating with not only your child but also his teacher. Keep in mind that children dealing with ADHD tend to respond positively to positive reinforcements and specific goals. The behavioral plan should also consist of the rewards that they deserve.

This means that there are instances when you need to create a chart where you can post stars in case he behaves well in class. This should serve as his source of motivation. The behavior plan should also be developed in such a way that your child will have minor rewards in case of small victories as well as big rewards in case he accomplishes something big.

The behavior plan should also consist of routines that he needs to follow at home. This is the key to supporting his journey towards lowering his risk of misbehaving in school. One important routine is to set a schedule for his homework. Schedule his homework at the same time daily. There should also be a specific spot for him to do his homework.

Do not forget to have a 10- to 20-minute break, giving him the chance to move away from the homework. Each break should not involve the use of a phone, TV, or any gadget, though.

Another tip when creating routines is to make a calendar that he can use in monitoring his assignments. Create a method that he can use in figuring out which among his assignments should be prioritized.

For instance, you can implement the color-coding scheme to give him an idea about prioritizing. He is even allowed to utilize an app as a means of organizing his assignments and tasks and managing time. The following can also be a big help to your child in retaining his focus, especially when trying to organize and complete his assignments:

- **Clutter-free workspace** – Note that he needs a workspace free of clutter and distraction to be able to focus. If possible, this space should be close to an adult. This is to ensure that someone is always around to guide him in maintaining his focus. Eliminate all sorts of distractions, too, including screens and gadgets.

- **Whiteboard calendar** – Your home should also have a visible and large whiteboard calendar where you can write and transfer his long-term projects and assignments. With this around, he can keep track of his tasks more effectively because he can see them.

- **Parent and teacher daily communication log** – This can benefit you the most as it gives you the chance to work more effectively together with his teacher. This is a big help in finding more effective solutions for him to learn.

Aside from that, remember that you can expect your child to retain his focus not only in school but also at home if you create a schedule for him before and after class when he can move and be active.

Students with ADHD may become so easily distracted by noises, passersby, or their thoughts that they often miss vital classroom information. These children have trouble staying focused on tasks that require sustained mental effort. They may seem as if they're listening to you, but something tends to get in the way of their ability to retain the information.

Find ways to deal with his distractibility

One common symptom of ADHD that can greatly affect your child in school is his distractibility. If your child seems to get distracted easily because of his disorder then there are ways to handle this symptom, including physical placement, breaking long work stretches into shorter and manageable chunks, and increased movement. In class, make sure that his seat is not close to the windows and doors.

When at home, eliminate all sources of distractions for him each time he needs to complete a school project or assignment. For instance, you may want to put your pet in a corner or another room – one that your child can't see and easily access. Managing distractibility is also possible by alternating those activities that require him to be seated with the ones that let him move around the classroom.

If possible, ask the teacher to include physical movements in class. Another thing to avoid distractibility is to write down all vital information in a spot where he can easily and effortlessly reference and read. Continue reminding him of the exact spot where he can find such information.

Large tasks and assignments should also be divided into smaller chunks so your child will have a chance to take a break from time to time. This will prevent him from getting bored, which might only cause him to get distracted even more quickly.

Manage his tendency to interrupt

ADHD makes it hard for your child to control his impulses, causing him to speak out in class even if it is not his turn yet or interrupt the talk of others. In class, he might comment or call out even if other people around him are still talking. The problem with these interruptions and outbursts is that others might see these as rude and aggressive, creating social issues.

What makes it even worse is that pointing out the problem can hurt your child's fragile self-esteem, especially if he is called out in front of the class or other family members. This is the main reason why you should correct his interruptions carefully. Your goal is to maintain his self-esteem as much as possible.

Try to communicate with his teacher and request for a more effective means of correcting such behavior without having to do it in front of others. You may want to create a secret language that only you and your child can understand. It could be in the form of discreet words and gestures that will let him know right away if he starts interrupting others.

Let his teachers know about this secret language, too, so they can use it in managing your child when he displays the behavior. Do not forget to praise your child every time he was able to complete a day successfully without interrupting conversations.

Teach him how to curb his impulses

The impulses of kids with ADHD are often so strong, causing social situations harder to deal with, especially if you pair it up with all the problems they experience inside the class. Due to their inability to control their impulses, others may find them unruly or aggressive. Your child's impulsivity, therefore, is one of his most troublesome ADHD symptoms, especially in school.

The most effective ways to manage your child's impulsivity include using behavior plans, implementing discipline in case of violations of some rules you have set up, and creating a plan designed to provide him with a sense of control over his impulses throughout the day. These simple tips are also helpful:

- Write down a behavior plan and put it close to him – A wise advice is to tape this plan into his desk or wall. This will allow him to see it all the time.

- Inform him about the consequences of his actions – Discipline him by letting him know about the consequences that he have to deal with in case he misbehaves. If possible, give the consequence right after misbehaving. However, make sure that you also clearly and specifically explain what went wrong. Your child should know what he did exactly so he can prevent himself from doing it again in the future.

- Reward him for good behavior – If he did a great job in fighting and controlling his impulses, then make sure to recognize his effort. Praise him aloud but make sure that you to tell him what it is specifically that he did correctly. This will encourage him to do things the right way.

- Create a daily schedule for him – Put it in writing. Write his schedule on paper or board then cross off each completed task. Note that this is a major help in gaining a sense of control even with his impulsivity. Knowing exactly what he should expect during the day, especially when he is at school, can calm him down, thereby preventing him from becoming too impulsive.

Minimize hyperactivity and fidgeting

Another major ADHD symptom is hyperactivity, causing your child to be in physical motion constantly. Because of his hyperactivity, you will find him struggling to stay in his seat. It is even possible for him to do extreme physical movements while in class, like twisting, kicking, jumping, and fidgeting. He may also move in such a way that his teachers will have an extremely hard time teaching him.

To fight hyperactivity in your ADHD-afflicted child, you need to look for creative solutions that will let him move appropriately and at the right time. Make sure to release his energy appropriately so he can calm down once his classes start. One of the things that you can do is to let him do an errand or task for you before going to school.

It could be as simple as letting him walk across the house to put away and wash dishes or sharpen his pencils. Another nice solution is to motivate him to get involved in sports. You may also encourage him to run before and after his classes. Furthermore, make sure that he does not miss his physical education classes and mealtimes.

You can also give him a small toy, stress ball, or any other object he can play with or squeeze discreetly while he is on his seat. Moreover, it is important to limit his use of the gadget. Reduce screen time as much as possible so he can replace it with more movements during breaks. This is a good way to lessen his excessive amounts of energy, making him relax once it is time for class.

Train him to follow directions

Another symptom of ADHD-afflicted kids that might cause problems at school is the inability to follow instructions/directions. You may find some of them looking like they clearly understood the directions. There are even instances when they write those down. The problem is they can't seem to follow once the teachers start asking them. This results in them missing some steps and submitting incomplete work.

They are also at risk of fully misunderstanding their assigned tasks, causing them to make something entirely different from what is asked. To train your child to follow instructions, try to break down the involved steps and instructions in a particular task, and reinforce them. If necessary, redirect each step and instruction, too.

You can do that by shortening the instructions. Keep each step as brief, simple, and easy to understand as possible. By doing that, he can complete each step without the hassle and figure out what he should do next. Remind him calmly each time he seems to lose direction.

Use a calm and firm voice when redirecting him to the right path.

You may also want to write down directions using colored chalk or bold marker on a blackboard or whiteboard. Make it as visible and accessible to him as possible.

Make the learning experience as fun and exciting as possible

Work with your child's teacher to make the learning process fun and exciting for him. Note that because of his disorder, your child is prone to losing focus easily. He might get bored if he does not see something interesting while in class. With that in mind, you have to make the learning process fun and enjoyable for him to retain his focus.

Each lesson should involve physical motion from time to time. Connect somewhat dry and boring facts to exciting trivia. You may also want to invent fun songs to help your child remember details with ease while also enjoying the whole process of learning and lessening ADHD symptoms associated with lack of focus.

Another thing to remember is that most of those who have ADHD think concretely. They usually prefer touching, holding, or participating in a fun experience when learning something. For the math subject, for instance, it would be a big help for teachers and parents to use objects and games as a means of demonstrating math concepts. If he finds math boring then using the mentioned items will turn it into a fun and meaningful subject for him.

Among the things that you can use to play games are dominoes, dice, and memory cards. These are useful in making numbers and figures fun for him. Drawing pictures is also a big help, especially when you are trying to help him solve word problems. By giving illustrations, your child will be able to gain a full understanding of vital math concepts.

You can also train your child to love reading. Note that while reading is a skill where a lot of kids with ADHD struggle, you can lessen your child's difficulties in that area by making the learning process fun and exciting for him. You can do that by incorporating exciting and interesting stories and info when letting him read.

Make the whole session quality and cozy time, too. If possible, pick a story that you can act out. Allow your child to pick his character. Let him assign a character to you, too. Bring the story to life through costumes and by using funny and exaggerated voices.

Let him master the process of doing homework

Each time homework is assigned to your ADHD-afflicted child, use it as an opportunity to bond with him and teach him some of the things that will let him thrive well at school and any other learning environment. The good thing about homework is that it gives you the chance to offer support to your child directly as it is academic work that he has to do out of the classroom.

Use this chance to guide your child in succeeding at school by teaching him at a place where you and he feel extreme comfort – your home. Another advantage of having homework is that aside from helping him learn by writing some essays or solving math or arithmetic problems, it can also boost his study and organizational skills that are useful in thriving in class even with the disorder.

Note that while it is important for you to teach your child the value of the organization and how to understand certain concepts, you still have to let him know that his homework has to be accomplished in one evening because it has a deadline. With that, train him to turn in assignments and homework on time. You can help your child in such a case by giving him a constant structure.

One tip is to choose a certain spot and schedule for doing the homework. Ensure that the spot is devoid of any gadget, TV, clutter, or any other distractions, like pets and foods. Do not forget to give him a break as frequently as possible. It could be in 10- to 20-minute increments. Make him understand the importance of time.

In such a case, you can utilize timers and analog clocks to keep track of his efficiency when trying to finish his homework. Also, communicate with his teacher so the school will be of help in establishing the best homework set up for him – that is a consistent schedule and place for him to turn in his work without hassle.

Help improve his organization skills

You may think that it is extremely difficult for your child to stay organized due to his condition but it is possible. In terms of trying to help in boosting his organization skills, make sure to have a fresh start. This means that even if the school year already started, you may want to shop with him and choose some school supplies, including color-coded dividers, a 3-ring binders, and folders.

Be of assistance to your child in filing papers using the new organizational system that you introduce to him. For instance, you may want to introduce to him a system involving the use of a homework folder where he needs to file each of his completed assignments. You may also want to use color-coding folders in organizing any loose papers. Teach him the basics of filing appropriately.

Another thing that you can do to boost his organizational skills that will be of great help at school is to guide him in organizing his items every day. These include the contents of his pockets, backpack, and folders. As much as possible, store an additional set of school materials and textbooks at home.

He can use these things to practice his organizational skills even further. Furthermore, you may want to start teaching him how to create his checklist and use it. Allow him to cross each item that he has already completed from the checklist.

Know how your child wants to learn exactly

Try to gather as much information about what your child likes as far as learning is concerned. Note that if you supply him with info based on the specific method that allows him to absorb everything you throw at him with ease, then he will be able to view the whole learning process as fun and exciting. This is the main reason why you have to observe your child. Find out and understand the specific method that will allow him to learn the most.

By understanding that, it would be easier for you to help his teachers craft exciting lessons that are sure to provide him with lots of information. For instance, you may notice that he is more of an auditory learner. This means that he seems to learn the most via listening and talking. If that is the case, then one way to let him learn is reciting facts to the tune of his favorite music.

Another method is allowing them to play the role of someone who is talking on a radio show. Furthermore, you should let him work with his peers more frequently since he is someone who loves to talk and listen. There are also what we call visual learners, who tend to learn the most if they read or observe.

If you notice that your child is a visual learner then you may want to let him enjoy using various fonts on the PC when studying. Using flashcards with colors can also help him study more efficiently. It is also advisable to let him draw or write his ideas on paper. Your child may also belong to the group of learners known as tactile.

Tactile learners seem to gain more knowledge if there is movement or physical touch involved in a lesson. If your child is that way, it helps to supply jellybeans for counters as well as costumes to play the role of some vital parts of history and literature. Another learning method for tactile learners is collage-making. You may also want him to use clay.

Aside from all the tips mentioned in this specific section of the book regarding how to manage your child with ADHD once he is at school, it is also essential to communicate with his teacher often. Ask his teacher to talk to you from time to time so you can discuss the progress of your child.

Request his update from time to time so you will know the exact status of your child at school. You may want to use a folder that you can give to him and vice versa so the two of you can share notes and communicate regarding your ADHD-afflicted child's progress.

Managing Social Life

With the hyperactivity, distractibility, and impulsivity of your child suffering from ADHD, finding friends, socializing, and maintaining good relationships with his peers can be hard for him. However, he must overcome all the problems linked to managing his social life as building positive relationships with peers and meeting friends are among those that are important for kids.

Unfortunately, because of your child's condition, he may find it difficult to make and keep friends. It will also be hard for him to gain the acceptance of a large peer group. With that in mind, it is safe to say that the symptoms of ADHD tend ruining the attempts of your child to reach out to others through positive means.

It might make him feel alone, unlikeable, different, and isolated, especially if no one seems to welcome him into their group. This could be a truly painful experience for your child, which will have long-lasting effects.

If you want your child to start making friends and avoid the negative effects when an ADHD-afflicted kid tries to make friends with others, then you can rest assured that you, as his parent, can be of great help. It is now possible to help him by honing his social skills and capabilities. Here are the things you can do to achieve that.

- **Get a clear idea of the actual social problem** – Make sure to discuss the social issues your child is experiencing, especially at school. Your goal is to have an open and honest discussion so you will gain a full understanding of the exact and specific nature of social issues he is dealing with. For instance, it could be that he tends to lash out to other kids at school physically each time they call him names.

Once you have a clear idea of the problem, make sure to acknowledge the unwanted and bad feelings that come with it. This means letting him know that feeling upset due to being teased is normal. However, you also have to figure out a way to tell him gently yet firmly that there are other better ways to respond to teasing than violence.

- **Discuss and rehearse some acceptable ways to respond** – Keep in mind that it is a bit hard to recognize ADHD in children. This is especially true when they are with their peers, making them prone to wrong misinterpretations. This is mainly because the way they communicate is different from other normal kids. The difference may confuse their peers.

If you have a child with ADHD, therefore, then look for a way to train them about some of the acceptable alternative responses to harsh and rude remarks and teasing. Let him know that there are several responses to teasing – some are good while the others are quite bad. Let him know that responding through physical violence, like shoving or punching his peers is an extremely bad idea.

One good alternative response involves simply walking away. He could also directly tell his peers to stop what they are doing without laying his hands on them. This will let him have control over the situation without showing aggressive behaviors. It would also be best to train him to maintain eye contact paired with a calm and relaxed body demeanor.

- **Motivate your child to write a journal regarding social interactions** – When journaling, ask him to clearly describe what he feels when interacting with his peers and in any other social setting. Let him write about what he thinks he did well when interacting with others. Also, encourage him to be honest when journaling.

For instance, let him write about the things that he should have done differently during the day he was at school or in any other social situation.

If he misbehaved, find out exactly how such behavior made an impact on his peer through the journal. What is great about this activity is that it helps in improving his written expression. It also boosts his sensitivity to others while also building his awareness of feelings and emotions.

- **Keep track of his social interactions actively** – Ensure that you play an active role in monitoring the social interactions of your child, especially at school. This helps in preventing painful misunderstandings and negative interactions with peers.

For instance, you can prevent your child from misinterpreting a situation, like when he thinks that a peer no longer wants to be friends with him just because he was unable to convince him to play outside. If that is the case, then you can provide him with possible reasons why his friend does not want to do what he wants.

It could be because he is busy doing other things, like finishing his homework or taking care of his sister. By playing an active part in his social interactions, you can supply him with possibilities and reasons for a specific situation, thereby preventing misunderstandings.

- **Boost his social awareness** – Because of his disorder, your child might also poorly monitor his social behaviors. It is because having ADHD makes it harder for him to gain full awareness and a clear understanding of social situations as well as the specific reactions he tends to incite in others. For instance, he may wrongly assume that his interaction with his classmate went smoothly when it was clear that it did not.

    It is mainly because the difficulties and challenges related to ADHD can lead to his weakened ability to read or assess a social situation accurately. He might also have a hard time self-monitoring, self-evaluating, and adjusting in a social situation when necessary. You need to focus on boosting his social awareness by teaching him the mentioned skills directly.

- **Teach your child social skills directly** – Train your child on how to interact with others and behave properly in a social setting. Do not forget to practice the skills you have taught him so he can hone those. Note that kids suffering from ADHD find it difficult to learn from their experiences in the past, causing them to react and respond without carefully thinking about the consequences.

One effective method of directly training and honing your child's social skills is to give them frequent and immediate feedback regarding their social miscues and unwanted and inappropriate behaviors. You can practice, model, and train him with positive social skills through role-playing. It is also a great way to teach him the best way to respond to and handle challenging social situations, such as teasing.

You can begin the whole training session by targeting one to two areas where your child struggles the most. By doing that, the learning process will not become extremely overwhelming and difficult for him. Some kids diagnosed with ADHD have a hard time learning the basics of socialization, such as starting a conversation and maintaining it and interacting with others reciprocally (ex. talking, listening, asking the feelings and ideas of the one they are talking to, displaying their interest in others, and taking turns when talking.

These kids may also find it hard to negotiate and resolve conflicts, maintain and share personal space, and speak using a normal tone (not an extremely loud one). If you notice that your child is one of those ADHD-afflicted kids who struggle with the basics, then give him clear details and info about acceptable social behaviors and rules.

Make it a point to practice these positive social skills repeatedly. It also helps to give immediate rewards to shape any positive behaviors and skills he has developed.

- **Build opportunities for your child to establish friendships** – As a parent, you should also be responsible for creating opportunities for your ADHD-diagnosed child to meet new friends. For instance, if he is either in pre-school or elementary then you can schedule playdates with one to two friends. It would be ideal to keep the circle small at first, instead of inviting a huge group instantly.

Scheduling a playtime for them can give you the chance to coach your child and model some positive ways to interact with peers. It is also a great way to practice the skills you have taught him. Make sure to structure this playtime in such a way that your child will be successful in interacting with his friends.

Consider yourself as the friendship coach of your child. Think carefully about how long you can hold the playdate with your child not acting up. Pick activities carefully. Go for those that your child will find fun, entertaining, and interesting. As he gets older, though, you will realize that building friendships and peer relationships become more complex and difficult.

Despite that, it is still important for you to get yourself involved in the process. Continue facilitating positive interactions with his peers. Also, remember that the middle and high school years are among the hardest periods of your child's life because he will most likely struggle during this time socially.

It would be ideal for him to have at least one trusted friend by his side during this time. It can already make him feel protected from the harsh effects of being ostracized by his peer group in case they reject him. However, because of the repeated rejection and social isolation, your child might also be at risk of desperately seeking the company of someone, even from one who can be considered as a bad influence.

With that in mind, you have to continue trying to give him opportunities for social interactions that will have a positive influence on him. For instance, you can start researching and participating in groups fostering positive social skills and peer relationships. You can get your child involved in groups, like Boy Scouts, Girl Scouts, or any sports team.

Just make sure that you give a sort of background about ADHD to the coach or group leader. By being familiar with the condition, the coach or leader will be able to work with you to create a more positive and supportive environment for your child designed to hone his pro-social skills.

Also, it is advisable to get in touch with his coach, the school, and some parents in the neighborhood. This will give you an idea about the things that your child goes through as well as whom he spends the most time with. Keep in mind that the peer group of your child and the traits of the group in its entirety can strongly influence your child. This is the main reason why you have to play an active role in building opportunities for him to establish friendships.

- **Improve the peer status of your child by reaching out to his school** – Note that once the peer group of your child labels him negatively due to his lack of social skills, dispelling the reputation will be extremely hard. The problem is that this negative reputation is the biggest hurdle that he might need to survive socially.

However, a child with ADHD might already establish his negative status in a peer group during early to middle school years, causing such status to stick even as he starts taking steps to change and improve his social skills. This is the main reason why you need to reach out to his teachers and coaches. Your goal here is to work with the school officials to address the effects of your child's reputation on his social life.

One thing that you can do is to build a positive and strong working relationship with his teachers. Give his teachers a clear idea about the strengths of your child, as well as his interests and struggles. Provide solutions that you noticed are extremely helpful when it comes to dealing with the weaknesses of your child.

Also, remember that most kids observe their teachers when trying to form social views about those who are part of their peer group. This is the main reason why the gentle redirection, acceptance, patience, support, and warmth of your child's teachers play a huge role in his social status.

If your child dealt with failures in class then the role of his teacher becomes even more important. It is because it is the role of his teacher to find conscious ways in attracting positive attention and interest to him despite his failures.

One strategy that the teacher can implement is to give special responsibilities and tasks to your child while the other kids in the class are present.

Ensure that the assigned responsibilities are those that your child has a higher chance of success. These should help him build a sense of self-acceptance and self-worth in class. This is a great way to offer opportunities for the members of his peer group to perceive your child positively. It also helps in stopping peer rejection.

Another thing that you can suggest to his teacher is to pair him up with a buddy who is compassionate enough to accept him. This is a huge help in facilitating social acceptance. It is also advisable to collaborate and communicate with his teacher constantly so you will gain an assurance that the class environment is indeed friendly to those dealing with ADHD.

By assuring you that, managing the symptoms of ADHD will be much easier for your child. Collaborating with his coach, teacher, or any other adult caregiver in school to implement the most effective social skills training and behavioral management approaches is also essential.

If your child needs to take medications then make sure that he is doing so on time. Note that his medications can contribute a lot in lessening his negative behaviors, especially those that his peers consider as rude, off-putting, and annoying. Work collaboratively and closely with his doctor to ensure that his medication is updated and correct.

Remember that for his medication to maximize its benefits in managing and fighting the core symptoms of the disorder, it is crucial to fine-tune, keep track of, and do some necessary adjustments on an ongoing basis.

- **Address specific social challenges** – Another way to help your child manage social situations more effectively is to learn about the specific social challenges he experiences and address them. You have to craft solutions based on the specific challenge your child is dealing with. For example, there may be times when he experiences difficulties maintaining and keeping friendships.

It could be because some ADHD-afflicted kids are too demanding and intense without them being aware of it. It might be difficult for them to take turns and share, causing their friendships and relationships to suffer. If your child experiences that, then maybe it is time to sign him up for a group or sports activity.

It is because it has been discovered that those dealing with ADHD find it easier to learn and understand the value of give-and-take when they are in a group, instead of in a one-on-one setting. Another common social challenge that ADHD patients have is their tendency to go off-topic.

It is because they are prone to losing track of a particular conversation or have some unrelated thoughts that distract them. There is also a high chance for them to misinterpret or misunderstand the things that other people say to them. To help him with that particular issue, you may want to record some conversations.

You should then encourage him to listen to the recorded conversation then discuss the specific times when both of you heard someone who tends to go off-topic. After identifying that, you can begin discussing ways that could have been done to improve the conversation. With that, your child will have an idea about what he should do next to avoid straying away from the topic.

Your child's ADHD might also cause him to be unreliable, which might harm his friendship and relationship with other people. This unreliability is characterized by troubles creating a plan, sticking to it, and following through. Because of that, those around him might start believing that they can't count on him whenever they are together in a group project.

If you noticed that this is the problem of your child then encourage him to talk to his group members about delegating tasks. You should then offer your assistance in creating a chart or checklist so he can monitor his progress. Another potential problem of your child in a social setting is his tendency to overreact.

Your child may find it difficult to manage his emotions, causing him to lash out each time he gets upset or have meltdowns even if his age is no longer appropriate for that behavior. To help him in that particular challenge, make it a point to observe his feelings and emotions, such as irritation and anger.

Train him to master his feelings and emotions, too. By teaching him to be mindful of what he feels exactly, it would be much easier for him to recognize every time his emotions are on a rise.

Managing the social life of your ADHD-afflicted kid should focus on boosting proper behaviors when in a social setting and reducing inappropriate ones. By training him in those appropriate behaviors and social skills, he can carry them over to other scenarios and situations that will have a positive impact on his quality of life. It is also necessary to make him understand how his actions influence and affect his environment.

Furthermore, teach him empathy to help him resolve conflicts and respect the rights and opinions of others. Teach him some basic social skills, such as apologizing, politeness, and greetings, too.

Chapter 4 – Medications for ADHD

While you can't still find an exact treatment for ADHD, various medications are available to improve the way your child functions and lessen his symptoms. Among the treatments that he can try are medication, training or education, psychotherapy, or combined recommended treatments.

Some of the medications that ADHD-afflicted children can safely take are those meant to lessen their impulsivity, distractibility, and hyperactivity. These medications are designed in such a way that they can help improve your child's ability to learn, work, and focus. Some of these can even boost their physical coordination.

However, be prepared to try a few medications and dosages to determine which one will work safely and effectively for your child. It is also important to let your child take medications only if his prescribing doctor carefully and closely monitors him.

Stimulant Medications

Among the medications that your child can take are stimulants or those products containing amphetamine and methylphenidate. These are the most commonly prescribed to ADHD sufferers. What is good about these stimulants is that they can boost and balance the levels of neurotransmitters that are considered as brain chemicals designed to help improve brain function.

Stimulants can also increase norepinephrine and dopamine – both of which are brain chemicals designed to play vital roles in attention and thinking. In most cases, stimulants are safe to take provided the intake is under the supervision of a medical professional. However, note that they also come with a few side effects and risks, especially if your child misuses it or takes more than the prescribed dosage.

In such cases, it might cause side effects like increased anxiety, heart rate, and blood pressure. You need to talk to the prescribing doctor if your child shows some side effects from taking the stimulant, including:

- Reduced appetite
- Increased irritability and anxiety

- Sleep problems
- Some changes in personality
- Tics characterized by sudden and repetitive sounds and movements
- Headaches
- Stomachaches

It is also necessary to set some precautionary measures in place before you begin giving your child stimulants or any other prescribed ADHD medication. For instance, ensure that he is taking the right dose and the correct medication prescribed by the doctor. It is a must to visit the doctor regularly, too, to figure out if there are any adjustments in the medication that you need to make.

If you are concerned about your child misusing or abusing the stimulants prescribed to him, then avoid making him in charge of taking it. Do not let him take the medicine without proper supervision. Lock the stimulant in a childproof container at home and put it in a place that your child can't easily reach.

This will prevent him from taking the medicine without your supervision and overdosing from it that might cause potentially fatal and serious consequences. Furthermore, you should avoid letting your child bring medications with him to school. It would be best to send it yourself and deliver it to the health office or the school nurse.

Non-stimulant Medications

Some non-stimulants can still be expected to help manage the symptoms of ADHD. While these non-stimulants seem to need more time to take effect in comparison to stimulants, you can still expect them to help boost attention and focus and minimize impulsivity.

Your child's doctor might prescribe a reliable non-stimulant in case he suffers from bothersome side effects when taking stimulants. Among the non-stimulants that work for ADHD, sufferers are atomoxetine, and some antidepressants, like bupropion.

Psychotherapy

Some psychotherapy and psychosocial interventions are also helpful for patients, as well as their loved ones when it comes to managing the signs and symptoms of ADHD and boosting their daily function. Also referred to as psychological counseling, the whole psychotherapy approach aims to educate you and your child about the disorder and hone some important learning and life skills that will help him succeed.

Among the things that psychotherapy can do for your child are:

- Improves organizational and time management skills
- Learns the basics of managing impulsive behaviors
- Hones problem-solving skills
- Improves self-esteem
- Recovers from social, work, and academic failures in the past
- Improves relationships with family, friends, and co-workers
- Learns some strategies to gain full control of temper

The different types of psychotherapy and psychosocial interventions that can produce such benefits for your child are the following:

- **Behavioral therapy** – The main goal of this form of psychotherapy is to help make some positive changes in your child's behavior. It often provides practical assistance, like in task organization, schoolwork completion, and handling difficult and emotionally draining situations. Through behavioral therapy, your child will be trained to monitor his behavior.

In most cases, it involves praising or rewarding him if he acts or behaves favorably, like when he was able to control his anger or think before he acts. When letting your child undergo behavioral therapy, it is not only you, as his parent, who can give insights regarding his behaviors.

Other family members, as well as his teachers, also have the authority to provide negative or positive feedback for specific behaviors and develop a clear list of chores, rules, and any other structured routines. All these are important in guiding your child to learn the basics of controlling his behavior.

The behavioral therapist you hired for your child will also most likely teach him basic social skills, like sharing toys or food, waiting for his turn, positively responding to teasing, and asking for help. The social skills training may also include learning appropriate responses to certain situations, reading facial expressions, and assessing other people's tone of voice.

- **Cognitive-behavioral therapy** – CBT also teaches your child some effective meditation and mindfulness techniques. It is a structured form of counseling, which hones his specific skills, especially in behavioral management as well as changing negative thoughts into positive ones.

  Through CBT, your child will be more aware of his situation and accept his feelings and thoughts. This acceptance can contribute a lot in boosting his concentration and focus. Your chosen cognitive behavioral therapist will also be the one to encourage your child to adjust to the changes that he might experience once he starts to undergo the treatment.

  These include thinking carefully before behaving in a certain way and resisting the temptation or urge to take risks unnecessarily. CBT is also a huge help in handling life challenges that your child might suffer at school, work, or when building relationships. Furthermore, this therapy can contribute to addressing other mental health problems, like substance misuse, anxiety, and depression.

- **Marital and family therapy** – It is important to note that your child is not the only one who should undergo therapy. Remember that parenting or taking care of a child with ADHD can be totally stressful and emotionally draining, so it also helps if you, your spouse, and the whole family involved in taking care of your child undergo a form of therapy – one of which is the marital and family therapy.

  Through this kind of therapy, you, your spouse, and other family members will be trained to deal with your child's disruptive behaviors. It also provides tips in encouraging behavioral changes and improving the way everyone interacts with your child.

- **Parenting skills training** – This form of training is also for parents of children suffering from ADHD. In this therapy, your skills in encouraging and rewarding positive behaviors will be honed. Here, you will get to know about various systems that will reward and implement consequences to change your child's disruptive behaviors.

  You will also be trained in providing positive and immediate feedback in case your child shows positive behaviors. It also helps you learn the basics of ignoring and redirecting unwanted behaviors as well as structuring situations in such a way that they start supporting favorable behaviors.

Alternative Medicines and Treatments

You may also want to try alternative medicines and treatments for your child. Remember that there is not that much research that shows how effective these alternative treatments are in lessening the symptoms of ADHD in children. However, it does not hurt to give them a try.

Before trying alternative medicines and interventions, discuss this plan with your doctor to figure out whether what you are thinking of using is safe. Among the safest alternative treatments you can try are:

- **Meditation or yoga** – What is good about meditation and various yoga routines is that they are meant for relaxation. This means doing them regularly can help your child relax. Both relaxation techniques can also teach your child the basics of discipline, helping him manage his ADHD symptoms effectively.

- **Special diets** – You can also try modifying the diet plans of your child. You can especially develop the diet plans in such a way that they promote positive benefits to ADHD-afflicted kits. A special diet for kids suffering from ADHD is that which does not contain foods that might raise their hyperactivity. These include foods containing sugar and common allergens, like eggs, milk, and wheat.

  Some ADHD-friendly diet plans also recommend staying away from foods containing additives and artificial food colorings. It is not also advisable to use caffeine as a stimulant for those suffering from ADHD because of its risky side effects.

- **Neuro-feedback training** – Also known as EEG (electroencephalographic) feedback, neuro-feedback training is also another alternative treatment that an ADHD patient can try. Each training session will let your child focus on specific tasks while utilizing a machine showing his brainwave patterns.

Coping and Proper Support

Taking care of a child suffering from ADHD is a major challenge not only for parents but also for the whole family. As a parent, you might get hurt each time your child misbehaves. You may also feel bad about how other people seem to respond to his misbehaviors. It can lead to stress that might eventually cause marital conflicts.

This is the main reason why everyone in the family, not just the child with ADHD, should learn some effective coping mechanisms and receive the proper support. It is also necessary to enjoy your time with your child. Exert an effort to appreciate and accept some parts of his personality that are good and not that difficult to deal with. Furthermore, you should strive to continue building healthy family relationships.

Conclusion

While challenging, having a child with ADHD is not that hard to deal with, so avoid losing hope. Continue believing in your child and his ability to cope. With proper support and the right form of treatment, it would be easier to control the symptoms of ADHD and create a life that he wants.

Also, remember that as his parent, you are the one who is responsible for giving him the treatment he needs. You will be the first one to take action and help him manage his symptoms. Fortunately, it is now easy to find the guidance you need, including health professionals, teachers, and therapists.

Furthermore, keep in mind that the key to finding the right treatment and coping mechanism for your child is to learn as much as you can about ADHD. By learning about this disorder, you can make informed and sound decisions that are extremely helpful in various aspects of your child's life and recovery.

CPSIA information can be obtained
at www.ICGtesting.com
Printed in the USA
BVHW051238051120
592612BV00014B/1704